T0383817

The Power of Parasites

Dalia Iskander

The Power of Parasites

Malaria as (un)conscious strategy

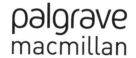

Dalia Iskander
Department of Anthropology
University College London
London, UK

ISBN 978-981-16-6763-3   ISBN 978-981-16-6764-0   (eBook)
https://doi.org/10.1007/978-981-16-6764-0

© The Editor(s) (if applicable) and The Author(s), under exclusive licence to Springer Nature Singapore Pte Ltd. 2021
This work is subject to copyright. All rights are solely and exclusively licensed by the Publisher, whether the whole or part of the material is concerned, specifically the rights of translation, reprinting, reuse of illustrations, recitation, broadcasting, reproduction on microfilms or in any other physical way, and transmission or information storage and retrieval, electronic adaptation, computer software, or by similar or dissimilar methodology now known or hereafter developed.
The use of general descriptive names, registered names, trademarks, service marks, etc. in this publication does not imply, even in the absence of a specific statement, that such names are exempt from the relevant protective laws and regulations and therefore free for general use.
The publisher, the authors and the editors are safe to assume that the advice and information in this book are believed to be true and accurate at the date of publication. Neither the publisher nor the authors or the editors give a warranty, expressed or implied, with respect to the material contained herein or for any errors or omissions that may have been made. The publisher remains neutral with regard to jurisdictional claims in published maps and institutional affiliations.

Cover image © Dalia Iskander

This Palgrave Macmillan imprint is published by the registered company Springer Nature Singapore Pte Ltd.
The registered company address is: 152 Beach Road, #21-01/04 Gateway East, Singapore 189721, Singapore

Acknowledgements

This book has been a long time in the making and relied upon the support, expertise and generosity of many organisations and people.

Above all, I owe a debt of gratitude to the people of Bataraza who opened up their homes, shared their food, made me laugh and imparted their experience, wisdom and knowledge. I will never forget how you gave up your time to talk to me and include me in parts of your lives. In particular, my thanks go to Danny, Ramil, Illaine, Bing, Dick, Babydan, Mary-Jane, Jerri, Kenneth, Kevin, Karily, Roderick, Edwin, Vilfred, Vangie, Aiza, Armelyn, Yolly, Riza, Patrick, Grace and all the staff and students at Matyag Elementary School, Taysay Elementary School, RVEMS and Saray Elementary School. The content and ideas expressed in this book came from all of you.

The doctoral work which forms the basis of this text would not have been possible without funding and resources made available by the UK Economic and Social Research Council, the Biosocial Society, the Parkes Foundation, the Royal Anthropological Institute, the Horniman Museum, PhotoVoice UK and the University of Durham. A network of academics and colleagues have provided guidance and support along the way and helped make my research possible: Kate Hampshire, Hannah Brown, Mark Booth, Effie Espino, Joy Lorenzo, Chris Drakeley, Clare Chandler, Steve Lindsey, Andrew Russell, Bob Simpson, Rebecca Marsland, James Spiller and Jessica Griffey, thank you.

In helping make this book happen, I am grateful to the team at Palgrave Macmillan (particularly Joshua Pitt and Sophie Lee) as well as the anonymous reviewers who helped get it published. Mohsin Zaidi, thank you for being an excellent (and easily distractible) writing companion. Ashraf Hoque, thank you for your helpful feedback on the proposal, advice on how not to do an index and your annual reminders for me to hurry up. I am grateful to Iris-Anne, Hugh and Annie for the use of their home for writing during a pandemic and to all the women at BT Nursery who helped take care of my daughter—their labour meant I could do mine. Emily Levitt, thank you for your careful reading, honest feedback and witty words of encouragement. And last but not least, to Charlie Cooper Henniker, you swept in and got me over the finish line with your eye for detail, literary flair and expert understanding of 'chilling'. I owe you an awful lot of pencils and all of my gratitude.

To my husband, daughter, family and friends, thank you—you'll be glad to know I'm done writing books.

Contents

1

Introduction

Malaria as Opportunity

It's early evening in mid-August, 2012. I have been in Bataraza for a week. I am with Ramil—a Tagbanua,[1] Pentecostal[2] pastor who has been living in Bataraza for many years. He is taking me to upland villages to meet people from the Pälawan community where malaria rates are highest according to records from the Rural Health Unit (RHU). From the main road that cuts through the centre of town, we begin to ascend the dirt tracks that weave through a mixture of secondary forest, cultivated fields and clusters of wooden nipa houses inhabited by mostly Pälawan families. After about an hour, we enter denser tree cover. The air feels cooler and the mosquitoes more abundant. Shortly after we arrive at a small cluster of houses, high in the forest, we take rest on the porch of a house belonging to Jimboy and his family who Ramil seems to know well. As Jimboy cuts open some fresh coconuts to quench our thirst, an old man approaches. He is slow on his feet, relying on a large stick he is carrying to keep him upright as he tra-

[1] The Tagbanua claim and are recognised by the government as being Indigenous to the central southern part of Palawan.

[2] The first Pentecostal missionaries arrived in the Philippines in the 1920s. Today, Evangelicalism is one of the minor Christian denominations comprising around 2% of the population according to the 2010 census.

© The Author(s), under exclusive license to Springer Nature Singapore Pte Ltd. 2021
D. Iskander, *The Power of Parasites*, https://doi.org/10.1007/978-981-16-6764-0_1

verses the dirt track. He looks tired and weak. He sits next to Ramil and, in hushed tones, whispers into his ear. Ramil listens sympathetically, nodding every now and then. The man stops and gestures in my direction in a way that suggests he is ushering Ramil to tell me something. Ramil duly informs me that the man has been suffering with a fever, headache, chills and body ache for three days and three nights. He saw us coming up the hill and came to ask if the 'American'[3] Ramil was with had any Paracetamol or money for him to buy some. The old man was speaking quietly in Palawano and I couldn't make out much of what he was saying. However, I was able to discern one word loud and clear, '*malarya*[4]'. Jimboy, handing me a freshly cut coconut and knowing I am interested in health, explains: 'We Pälawan have lived here since time immemorial. Our *kagurangurangan* (ancestors) are from this place. We have always had sicknesses like *bati*[5] and we know how to treat those from them. But *malarya* like this old man has, our *kagurangurangan* did not have that. If you want to know about the health of the people here, you must know about *malarya*.' I ask Ramil if we can take the man to the RHU or if we could contact a health worker to come to him in order to carry out a Rapid Diagnostic Test (RDT) for malaria. The man seems reluctant and soon leaves us. I express my concern to Ramil. 'He won't go the RHU'. He tells me. 'Four years ago, there was an outbreak of filariasis here and there were rumours that the health staff from the province were coming here to harm the people with drugs that came from America. The people here kept saying, "We don't want to die. We will not take your medicines". Don't worry Dalia. I know this man. He most probably doesn't have those parasites in his blood. But it's like that here, the IPs [Indigenous People] just need to say the word *malarya* and they can get things. *Malarya* is for them, how do you say in English, also an opportunity. He will get the help he needs.'

---

[3] It is not uncommon for Filipinos to refer to any foreigner as American and men are often called 'Joe' (as in GI Joe, a nickname for American soldiers during World War II).

[4] In this book, I use the English term 'malaria' to denote the disease as it is conceived in largely biomedical terms implying a specific aetiology, presentation and treatment in line with this medical system. For some participants, mainly health staff working in 'formal' healthcare settings (hospitals, clinics, etc.) as well some government leaders, this was what I gleaned they meant when they used the term. In contrast, I use the Tagalog term *malarya* to echo other participants' use of the word that denoted a broader illness category described throughout the book. There is of course overlap and the terms are somewhat interchangeable.

[5] *Bati* comes from *nabati* in Tagalog meaning to be greeted, or *salibegbeg/samban* in Palawano, and refers to sicknesses presenting in similar ways to malaria as discussed in Chaps. 3, 4, 5, and 6.

In the municipality of Bataraza on the Filipino island of Palawan, the fever, chills, headache, body ache and vomiting that are characteristic symptoms of the parasitic disease known across the world as malaria were common ailments among Pälawan communities living in the remote foothills. I never did find out if the old man I met that day did or did not have parasites in his blood, or what happened to him after our encounter, but our conversation stayed with me throughout my time on Palawan. It was my first interaction with someone who described their malady as *malarya* and, although I didn't realise it then, encapsulated the Janus-faced nature of the disease in this context. The parasites that Ramil referred to caused suffering and even death occasionally among Pälawan communities at the same time as they presented them with 'opportunities', including those potentially afforded by a newly arrived anthropologist. I would come to understand this ambivalence a little more during my time in Bataraza, and see for myself what drawbacks and benefits *malarya* was tied into for upland communities. It is this tension that I unpack in this book. I ask how and why it was that *malarya* both frustrated and facilitated life for the Indigenous Pälawan and what this tells us about the nature of the disease specifically as well as about social relations more broadly. I conclude that we cannot understand the power of parasites separate from the human relations that surround them. In fact, the two are so intertwined that by understanding human practices, we come to understand parasites, and by understanding parasites, we come to understand human practices. It is for this reason that malaria and human strategic practice fold in on each other with an array of effects.

This seemingly simple observation has profound effects on how diseases such as malaria are approached. For example, in many ways, human relations are often side-lined in global health initiatives to prevent and treat the ill-effects of malaria parasites. As Abimbola and Pai (2020) point out, global health emerged as an enabler of European colonisation and has since taken on different forms—colonial medicine, missionary medicine, tropical medicine and international health. Historical accounts of European infectious disease research in the expansionist era of the late nineteenth and early twentieth centuries (that formed the foundation of what is referred to today as global health) have largely focussed on describing the proliferation of ideas that come under the umbrella of what Anderson (2004) characterises as an 'arid waste of reductionism' (ibid., p. 41). In essence, these approaches were predicated on breaking down phenomena into sets of variables that offered the possibility of identifying cause and effect. In the case of what the Italians called '*mal' aria*' in the nineteenth century—spoiled air emanating from decomposing vegetation thought to be the source of fever—written history tells us that European scientific practices gradually overturned such thinking in professional circles by instead attributing fever to an effect caused by the occurrence of *Plasmodium* parasites in the body, passed to humans through bites from *Anopheles* mosquitoes (Cox, 2010). A series of scientific processes in microbiology have rendered the parasite visible to humans and, since then, malaria and *Plasmodium* have continued to collapse in on each other to the point that they are largely synonymous in global health arenas: parasites are malaria and malarias are parasites. The World Health Organization (2020a) (WHO) epitomises this in the seemingly benign definition it offers in its malaria 'fact sheet': 'Malaria is caused by *Plasmodium* parasites'.

Anderson (2004) points out that a focus on the parasite that began in nineteenth-century European scientific practice and still influences global health today did encompass a wider interest in the environmental conditions that allowed parasites to flourish. Although remaining on the margins, some European scientists went beyond mere 'microbe hunting' in trying to map out the factors that disrupted what they saw as the delicate ecological 'equilibrium' in which parasites, mosquitoes and humans lived (ibid.). In the arena of contemporary global health, practitioners trying to prevent or treat malaria the world over continue to take a wide variety of approaches and focus on different elements of the complex connections between parasites and their wider context including human action to some extent. From an epidemiological point of view this makes good sense: human malaria emerges out of a series of connections between parasites and two hosts—mosquitoes and humans. Five species of *Plasmodium* parasite are thought to cause illness in humans.[6] Within

---

[6] *Plasmodium falciparum, Plasmodium vivax, Plasmodium ovale, Plasmodium malariae* and *Plasmodium knowlesi.*

scientific frameworks, their lifecycle is complex and takes weeks to complete. Sexual stages of the parasite reproduce in the midgut of female *Anopheles* mosquitoes,[7] some migrating to the mosquitoes' salivary glands. As the adult female mosquito needs blood in order to produce fertile eggs, it seeks out hosts including humans to bite, inadvertently transmitting *Plasmodium* sporozoites (immature forms of the parasite) into the human bloodstream with their saliva. Once in the body, sporozoites that are not immediately destroyed by the immune system are taken up by liver cells, in which they mature and then rupture from in their thousands, by now in their next form—merozoites. Released into the bloodstream, they go undetected by the human body under the camouflage of liver cell membranes and begin attaching to red blood cells. As they replicate asexually inside, they cause cells to explode, releasing yet more merozoites that can attach to yet more red blood cells. This results in the characteristic cycles of fever and chills that typify human malaria. To complete their lifecycle, some differentiate into male and female forms of the parasite (gametocytes) that, if ingested back into a mosquito's midgut, can mate. After 10–18 days they are released again in the mosquito as sporozoites which, so long as ambient temperature in the gut is adequate and the mosquito lives long enough,[8] can be transmitted into a host in the insect's next bite. Thus, the cycle continues.

Given the complex web of relations needed to ensure their own survival, these parasites complete their lifecycle against the odds. When viewed within this framework, interrupting the transmission of the parasite in both mosquito and human hosts is a clear way to reduce infection. Lindsay et al. (2004) therefore describe how contemporary global health policy efforts to do so revolve around preventing the parasite lifecycle completing in the bodies of mosquitoes and humans through a range of strategies: environmental management initiatives are used to modify or manipulate landscapes in order to reduce their receptivity to mosquitoes; insecticides are used on breeding sites, and on nets, screens and lotions in

---

[7] According to the World Health Organization (2020a), there are more than 400 different species of *Anopheles* mosquito with around 30 characterised as malaria vectors of major importance.

[8] Adult female *Anopheles* live for an average of 10–14 days.

order to kill mosquitoes or discourage them from passing on parasites to humans; and vaccines and anti-malarial drugs are administered to human hosts to limit or interrupt the parasite load inside bodies. There is no doubt that these approaches have yielded significant results when it comes to reducing illness and death. The latest *World Malaria Report* from the WHO (2020b) suggests that in 2019, the incidence rate of malaria declined globally to 57 cases per 1000 population at risk, down from 80 in 2000. In addition, 27 countries reported fewer than 100 Indigenous cases and had thus moved to the 'elimination' stage. An estimated 1.5 billion malaria cases and 7.6 million malaria deaths were thought to have been averted in the period 2000–2019. Nevertheless, worldwide, there were an estimated 229 million cases of malaria and 409,000 reported deaths in 2019, 84% of which were among children aged under five, with the highest burden in Africa followed by Southeast Asia. The 'battle' against parasites that cause suffering, misery and death for so many thus continues.

However, in global health policy, when humans are specifically targeted for intervention to reduce cases of malaria, their behaviours tend to be interrogated in terms of their *response* to parasites and the extent to which they adhere to the prevention and treatment measures mentioned above. Although the environment in which parasites exist is taken into account by many, reductionism still remains to some extent: the idea that biological/natural/non-human phenomenon such as parasites exist as separate entities to social/cultural/human variation is still implicit. Another implication persists: that power—simply defined here as the capacity to take action (Haugaard, 2008, p. 194)—is considered only achievable at the expense of someone/something else's demise. The non-human world exerts its power *over* us in allowing disease to survive but we can respond in ways that ultimately exert our power back *over* it by 'avoiding', 'controlling', 'eliminating' or even 'eradicating' it in order to survive ourselves. Inherent here is the notion that parasites and people are locked in a sort of struggle to endure non-human on one side and human on the other. Power is embroiled in a zero-sum game in this formulation—the parasite *or* human harnesses power to take action at the expense of the other. Educating humans about parasites and how to modify their behaviour in order to evade, interrupt, or destroy their biological processes is therefore often framed as the human-orientated route to change in global health policy.

In this book I counter this impression and deal with human practice in a different manner, one opposed to the characterisation I have illustrated earlier. Instead, I address the way in which human practice and parasites are linked in specific contexts and suggest it is to such a profound extent that they do not exist independent from each other as stable entities with neatly distinct and discernible boundaries. The resulting implication of this assertion is that power becomes implicated in a more complex set of relations than those with simply zero-sum outcomes alone. The indelible and permeable link between parasites and humans seems to rest on a dynamic whereby reducing some of the power or agency of one does not necessarily always increase it in the other, and *vice versa*. The way power plays out in this intricate web of relations is complex and far from clear-cut. As the vignette above illustrates, the mutual relationship between parasites and human practice is so obscured that even when parasites are not necessarily 'in the blood' of a human host at all, as Ramil conjectured about the old man we met, they still have the ability to afford a certain kind of effect on humans and the actions they take. As such, malaria (even in its absence) provides an opportunity to trace the inextricable way in which the trajectory of humans and non-humans are entangled, or as Nading (2014) puts it in relation to dengue fever, how they co-exist as 'a heterogenous knot of connections that undermines simple spatial, social and species barriers' (ibid., p. 11).

Malaria and Anthropology

The assertion that malaria and practice are so deeply interrelated has implications for anthropology as well as global health policy. A focus on infectious diseases such as malaria is not new to the discipline. As Chandler and Beisel (2017) have documented, anthropologists have increasingly broken down boundaries between the biological and the social in the arena of malaria to the extent to which the social is no longer relegated to a set of 'determinants' of (a fixed) biological disease but actually implicated in its very making and the nature it takes. Conceiving of diseases as combined social, biological, material and semiotic processes in this way (Latour, 1988; Law, 2008) has yielded important insights. For example, authors such as Mol (2002) have argued that it is problematic to speak of one disease as if it were a singular, neutral and naturalised phenomenon. Rather, her theoretical assertion is that a multiplicity of diseases are created in specific contexts through the range of human practices that are enacted by individuals *in relationship* to other human actors and the non-human world, rather than in isolation. As individual experience does not exist in a vacuum, different practices and the multiple diseases they implicate often cohere through shared understandings and the act of employing strategies in coordination. It is for this reason that we can speak of and perform around 'malaria' as a singular, mutually intelligible disease across many different experiential, spatial and temporal domains, despite its multifarious nature.

Through focussing on the way malaria is enacted differently through practice, anthropologists have demonstrated how specific contours of the disease come into being in the hands of a range of human actors in defined contexts. For example, Eckl (2017) has argued that how malaria is defined, what kind of problem it poses, to whom it poses a problem, what solutions are advocated to deal with it and who the providers of these solutions are is not fixed. Rather, these interrelated factors are all open *to interpretative flexibility* by global policy 'experts' who negotiate various boundaries as they navigate malaria control's complex milieu of philanthropy, funding and politics. He demonstrated the impact of this through describing the way in which technical-biomedical solutions have increasingly prevailed over socio-medical ones in contemporary global health policy circles despite the long-standing awareness of the social and environmental dimensions of the disease throughout history, as alluded to above. He argues that universally applicable solutions have continued to be prioritised in these arenas over the acknowledgement of local variations of malaria and locally tailored solutions, again despite the latter having been consistently highlighted by various actors. As such, the universal, biomedical, technical malaria of contemporary global policy, largely instigated in European and North American contexts, seems a product of circumstance and uneven relations of power rather than of inevitability.

As well as policy-makers, anthropologists have similarly interrogated the practices of professionals who are responsible for managing malaria on the ground and here, too, emphasised the contingent nature of their seemingly 'neutral' techniques of dealing with malaria. For example, Chandler et al. (2012) demonstrated how clinicians in Yaoundé and Bamenda, Cameroon, enacted top-down policy guidelines in ways that were not simply driven by the presence of parasites *per se*. Instead, they used Rapid Diagnostic Tests (RDTs) and anti-malarial drugs in line with broader desires to meet the needs of their patients who themselves defined what constituted malaria and demanded what tests or treatments should be offered. For these practitioners, the use of technologies such as tests and medicines were bound up in their wider efforts to preserve their reputations as experts who could effectively deploy appropriate symbols of care in meeting their patients' psychological, economic and social requirements. Marsland (2007) furthermore showed how in attending to patients, practitioners acted in ways that blurred the boundaries between definitions and practices of 'biomedical' and 'traditional' disease. The 'hybrid' way that practitioners categorised and dealt with malaria in Kyela, Tanzania, was an intentional means to ensure their legitimacy and relevance as professionals. In the same vein, Kelly and Beisel (2011) showed how the practices of municipal workers responsible for applying insecticide to breeding grounds, quite literally in the back alleys of Dar es Salaam, also shaped what local malaria was and how it was tackled. Through deploying chemicals, community workers transformed local ecological conditions, simultaneously creating and attending to 'neglected' malarias that were obscured in grander policy activities. As they mapped the area in fine detail to conduct larval surveillance and monitoring, they defined and dealt with a malaria that was at a different spatial scale to that which was captured and targeted in large-scale mapping exercises. Paying similar attention to the local nature of malaria, Langwick (2007) argued that the actions of professionals intersected with patients and community members in Southern Tanzania in a manner that also shaped the param-eters and trajectories of different illnesses. In her case, she showed how the boundaries between *degedege* (Kiswahili for a 'traditional' malady that begins with a jerk or a start and progresses to the body becoming hot, foaming at the mouth and eyes rolling to the back of the head) and malaria were not self-evident but variously overlapped, constricted and broadened through strategic practice. This suggests that the malaria identified and dealt with by practitioners and patients on the ground is equally as interpretive as the one in the hands of policy-makers described above.

Together, these studies have highlighted how malaria's 'historical, sociological and political life … exceeds the moment of the parasitological exchange' (Kelly & Beisel, 2011, p. 72). In focussing on how human practice brings disease into being and shapes its very nature, they have blurred the lines between culture and nature illustrating how the two are created in relation to each other in localised settings. An associated body of work has taken this further by challenging the human exceptionalism of focussing on people by bringing non-human agents into sharper view (Haraway, 2008; Kirksey & Helmreich, 2010; Tsing, 2012). In the case of malaria, this has involved challenging the multispecies separation of humans versus mosquitoes, parasites, animal hosts and plants, instead highlighting their entanglement in enmeshed ecologies (Beisel, 2010, 2015; Hoffman, 2016). Rather than restricting the anthropological gaze to just people, they have incorporated descriptions of how the non-human world affects change. Posing a methodological challenge to anthropologists who conventionally access the inner worlds of people, multispecies perspectives have dealt with this by weaving in scientific accounts of non-human agency. For example, the observations by those in life sciences, entomology, veterinary science, immunology and microbiology that once *Plasmodium* is in gut of the mosquito, it lulls it into sedation making it less likely to feed or feed for shorter durations on hosts including humans (and therefore risk being swatted to death in the process). Conversely, once the parasite has had time to incubate and needs to be passed on to complete its cycle, it promotes persistent feeding (Cator et al., 2014; Wekesa et al., 1992). When transmitted to a human, the parasite brings on the fever and fatigue that renders the host so exhausted and sedentary that it is ripe for biting. Parasites also increase human attractiveness to mosquitoes through making changes to their bodily odour (Batista et al., 2014; Busula et al., 2017; Lacroix et al., 2005). This, combined with adaptations the parasite has undergone to cope with genetic modifications that have developed in humans to increase their own survival rates (e.g., the ability to still infect Duffy-negative individuals[9]) as well as to drug treatments designed to destroy them (Packard, 2014), illustrates how assertively parasites bring power into the equation. The staggering numbers of deaths that malaria still causes around the world are the most sobering of reminders. *Anopheles* mosquitoes too demonstrate behavioural (Govella et al., 2013) and genetic resilience (World Health Organization, 2018b) to the insecticides used by humans on breeding grounds, houses, nets and bodies designed to disrupt or kill them. Insecticide resistance has become so widespread that the majority of WHO member countries reported it to at least one insecticide in their major malaria vectors (ibid.). This global incidence is prevalent to the extent that some are calling for chemical-free untreated nets to be used instead as a response that takes account of the entangled nature of human and non-human trajectories (Okumu, 2020).

Multispecies perspectives in anthropology have also led scholars to put the plants used to treat malaria at the centre of analyses in explaining how the disease unfolds in particular circumstances. For example, Hsu (2006b) situates the extraction of *qinghaosu* (Artemisinin) from the traditional Chinese medicinal plant *qing hao* (the blue-green *hao*[10]), which is now the significant ingredient in first- and second-line global treatments, in the specific political context of the People's Republic of China of the 1960s and 1970s. She showed how its revolutionary 'discovery' and extraction from *Artemisia annua* (sweet wormwood) plants at once blurred and reinforced boundaries between 'modern' and 'traditional' medicinal knowledge and practice. Similarly, taking an explicitly posthuman approach by putting Cinchona plants from South America at the centre of things, the historian Roy (2017) showed how the extraction of

---

[9] As described by Popovici et al. (2020).

[10] In her work, Hsu (2006a) argues that although Artemisinin is found in three species of the genus Artemisia—*A. lancea, A. annua* and *A. apiacea*, the latter two were known to the Chinese in antiquity but easily confused with each other and both provided material for the herbal drug *qing hao* (blue-green *hao*). However, at least the eleventh-century Chinese scholars recognised the difference between the two species and advocated the use of *A. apiacea*, rather than *A. annua* for 'treating lingering heat in joints and bones' and 'exhaustion due to heat/fevers' (ibid.).

quinine—the mainstay of malaria treatment around the world until the early twentieth century—shaped the making and persistence of malaria as a specific diagnostic category throughout nineteenth-century colonial India with enduring consequences. By articulating how cure and disease go hand in hand, these authors emphasise that the concept of malaria as a self-contained, de-historized, de-contextualised disease is, yet again, destabilised.

Anthropological approaches have thus highlighted how a series of complex interactions evoke specific enactments and articulations of malaria (Langwick, 2007) that are not self-evident but emerge in particular temporal and spatial 'hotspots' (Brown & Kelly, 2014). They force us to think of ecological environments as places that are historically humanly mediated, not given or discovered, and as spaces of pathogenic possibility (ibid.) where disease is the relation of everything from parasites, insects, plants and humans to policies, diagnostic tests, needles, maps and discourses, all with porous and overlapping boundaries. This 'mixed way things happen' (Mitchell, 2002, p. 52) is crucial to Mitchell's (2002) analysis of how mechanised war, famine, dams, irrigation, industrial pesticide production, sugar cultivation and post-colonial independence movements (to name but a few societal and environmental factors) came together to bring about the malaria epidemic of the 1940s in Egypt. Such 'infrastructural thinking' makes the disproportional way diseases are spread and the harm they cause inseparable from the equally disproportionate way human social relations are organised. In this way, diseases are never apolitical but always intimately tied within unequal distributions of power (Parker & Allen, 2014) and inseparable from human practice.

Malaria and Practice

This entanglement between disease and the vast array of human practice is at the centre of this book. Following scholarship in medical anthropology, I use the term 'practice' in relation to what people do because it 'captures the emergent and contingent properties of people's activities in particular situations' (Cohn, 2014, p. 157) and crucially because it takes account of the way power is embodied in practice (Bourdieu, 1977). This is in contrast to the term 'behaviour' which is often used in global health arenas and has embedded within it the notion that discrete actions (health behaviours) arise *in response* to discrete phenomena (malaria parasites). Grounded in positivism and reductionism, as discussed above, these approaches run the risk of constituting 'behaviours' as something easily identifiable that can be abstracted and neutralised as an object of observation and analysis. Cohn (2014) describes how the health behaviour concept that has pervaded global and public health in recent years is derived from Euro-American health psychology, particularly since the mid-twentieth century. Early models that gained traction revolved around the assumption that people did what they did in regard to health as a result of rational deliberation and reasoning, giving primacy to cognitive motives and intentions (ibid., p. 158). For example, the 1950s saw the development of Knowledge, Attitude, and Practice (KAP) surveys which were grounded in the idea that knowledge was a prerequisite to the intentional performance of health-related behaviours. Inherent in these studies, which are still widely used today in global health circles, was an underlying assumption that there was a direct relationship between discrete elements of knowledge and action. Significantly, these studies suggested that by using interventions to change specific knowledge (i.e., through education), associated changes in specific behaviours would follow suit. Other psychological models developed around the same time elaborated in more detail upon additional cognitive factors that potentially affected behaviour and incorporated non-deliberate, non-reasoned or automatic cognitive reflexes—referred to as habits. These included the Theory of Reasoned Action (Ajzen & Fishbein, 1973) and the Health Belief Model (Hochbaum, 1956). Central to these was the idea that explicit knowledge and direct intentions alone were not enough to affect behaviour, as more implicit and indirect notions such as self-esteem and self-efficacy also affected people's ability to act in certain ways.

While adding to the multiplicity of potential inputs, these models and many other psychological theories relating to behaviour change that have been developed in more recent years[11] suffer similar shortcomings.

---

[11] Michie et al. (2005) found that health psychology theorists, health services researchers and health psychologists identified 33 psychological theories that informed health behaviour research.

Essentially, they hinge on a 'linear order that conceives of various psychological determinants, potentially modified by social norms and triggered by environment cues, which then determine someone's behaviour' (Cohn, 2014, p. 159). These approaches are highly individualistic as behaviour is posited as an 'outcome of an individual who is presented as the obvious focus of both the processes preceding behaviour and the agent of the behaviour itself' (ibid.). As a result, many health behaviour interventions are targeted at the level of changing individual consciousness. This has manifested in a great number of studies that aim to 'educate' and/or 'empower' individuals to think differently about specific and defined health issues (i.e., by altering knowledge) and/or change their perceived agency in affecting their discrete health behaviours (i.e., by increasing levels of self-awareness, self-esteem and self-efficacy). However, as Cohn (2014) points out, 'a great wave of research over the last two decades attempting to develop techniques and evidence of behavioural change has proved to have surprisingly limited success' (ibid., p. 157).

In order to add to this body of health-related scholarship, I move away from the idea of malaria-related behaviours as a distinct category of variables that consciously arise at an individual level in response to a single, fixed phenomenon (malaria) that itself can be easily identified, observed, measured and targeted. Instead, I take an anthropological approach that is concerned with describing the breadth of practices that people engage in, in a much wider context, to explore what role these knotted relations (Haraway, 2008) might actually have in shaping the nature of disease and *vice versa*. In doing so, I aim to incorporate the 'social, affective, material and interrelational features of human activity' (Cohn, 2014, p. 159) and show how it *enacts*, rather than responds to, malaria. When approached in this way, the implications for global health are that parasites and the power they have can no longer be seen as separate to the much wider complex human relations that surround them. In terms of interventions, to target human relations is to target parasites, and to target parasites is to target human relations.

To demonstrate my argument, I document the practices of various groups of people in Bataraza and what impact these had on the nature of malaria in this context, in particular in relation to Pälawan communities. As described above, a growing body of work has taken inspiration from

Mol's (2002) assertion that diseases are enacted through a range of overlapping and interrelated human practices. While she demonstrated *how* different groups (patients, pathologists, surgeons, radiologists, laboratory technologists in her case) in different settings acted in relation to each other as well as to a whole host of non-human actors to create multiplicities of disease (atherosclerosis) in ways that 'hung' together as one mutually intelligible entity, her study was confined to the domain of health/medicine and left out the wider context that situated these practices. There was no further interrogation of *why* it was that people engaged in various practices beyond an assumed desire to diagnose and treat atherosclerosis. We did not really get a sense of how or why various actions came to be routinised over time to the point of becoming quotidian. As such, we were left with an unanswered question about what the mechanisms are through which practices operated. Similarly, although Mol (2002) explained how some divergent practices were 'distributed' far enough away or 'left out' completely in favour of coordination to make the disease cohere, she failed to address why these distributions occurred in the first place and, significantly, the effects in terms of the implications on people's lives—in other words, the role of unequal power relations in determining the existence and outcome of 'interferences', as she called them, was overlooked.

To counter this, I describe the practices of various groups of people ranging from government officials to Pälawan patients to describe why they engaged in certain practices, what effect this has on the way multifarious malaria was enacted, why certain enactments were prioritised over others and what impact this had on what Pälawan people set to gain and lose as a result. Crucially, I draw on Bourdieu's (1977, 1990) work to add to the literature on human practice and its interrelation with disease as cited above in order to explicate the mechanisms through which actions were generated and to hone in on role of power in mediating them. I argue that the actors described in this book framed and dealt with malaria in different fields (e.g., local government offices, clinics, homes): 'social arenas endowed with a specific gravity and force that influence the actions and reactions of social actors' (Veenstra & Burnett, 2014, p. 189) who have tacitly agreed to take part in the game of social life. Within these fields, actors' practices appeared to be orientated towards the aim of acquiring an embodied 'feel for the game' (Bourdieu, 1990) or 'practical mastery' (ibid., p. 2) of how to act in ways that were taken-for-granted but still 'strategically' orientated towards gaining various kinds of skill or competence (whether it be economic, social, cultural or symbolic capital). They gained these skills as they were endowed with what is referred to as '*habitus*'.[12] *Habitus* denotes an overall orientation of the Heideggerian (1967) notion of being-in-the-world (Sweetman, 2003) or the 'social dispositions and beliefs acquired and stored by social actors over time as they move[d] through social space, encounter different people and fields and reason their way through complex situations' (Veenstra & Burnett, 2014, p. 192). Importantly, Bourdieu (1977) argued that actors did not build *habitus* through just conscious deliberation and evaluation about how they 'should' act in accordance with the clear-cut 'rules' of society or when confronted with a particular fixed phenomenon (e.g., malaria) in a certain field—faculties of the reflexive mind alone, in other words. Instead, an unconscious, practical, embodied, bodily know-how was also built over time through creativity, adaption and change as 'each agent, wittingly or unwittingly, willy nilly, [was] a producer and reproducer of objective meaning' (ibid., p. 79). In doing so, actors achieved what Bourdieu (1977) called '*doxa*': where the 'natural' became a self-evident competence that people had of their place in the world in 'a quasi-perfect correspondence between the objective order and subjective principles of organization' (ibid., p. 164). I take the unconscious to therefore operate as taken-for-granted bodily know-how that resided somewhat beyond people's conscious grasp. *Habitus* therefore provides a framework against which human practice unfolded—a kind of underlying grammar (Crossley, 2001) or base from which people derived a predisposition for social action (Haugaard, 2008). This points to the dual (un)conscious quality of human practice. As Akram (2013) notes, the unconscious is somewhat controversial in the social sciences, occupying as it does a problematic space of being an unobservable entity with very observable effects. As she argued, Bourdieu (1977, 1990) himself did not explicitly

---

[12] As Haugaard (2008) explains, the concept of *habitus* is found in the work of Émile Durkheim, Max Weber, Georg Simmel and Marcel Mauss in different ways but became a significant part of the sociological repertoire since the 1980s as they work Pierre Bourdieu became increasingly popular.

state his position on the unconscious but his intent was to highlight its importance (albeit hidden) in descriptions of what people were actually doing. This has methodological implications as I will outline below.

It is important to note that highlighting the unconscious elements of practice should not be seen as being overly deterministic—it does not deny people agency nor imply that they lack awareness, concentration, resolve or intent in the actions they take and the goals they aim to achieve as a result. Rather, it is a point of emphasis—an observation that a lot of what constitutes agentive practice unfolds without any necessary 'deliberate pursuit of coherence ... without any conscious concentration' (Bourdieu, 1977, p. 170) and, as such, does so largely incoherently or even unnoticed at times.[13] Importantly, reflexivity was not absent in Bourdieu's formulation of *habitus*—a point often missed by critics who accuse him of social determinism.[14] *Habitus* was not regarded as only the unconscious. Rather, reflexiveness, intentionality, habit and the unconscious were all said to operate alongside each other in agency, and did not necessarily cancel each other out (Akram, 2013, p. 57). This is obvious within Bourdieu's formulation of *habitus* when he made clear that the unconscious was not the same as habit, conceived of in behavioural psychology as an automatic cognitive reflex as described above. As Akram (2013) stresses, whilst *habitus* included habit, Bourdieu and Wacquant (1992) were insistent that the two terms were not interchangeable, leading to the statement by Bourdieu: 'I said *habitus* so as not to say habit' (ibid., p. 22). *Habitus* was therefore a much more complex formulation of the grammar that informed practice than a reductionist view of habit as non-deliberate, non-reasoned, automatic cognitive reflexes of the mind. *Habitus*, by contrast, was conceived of as *both* mental and corporeal; inherited and generative; individual and collective; contemporary and historical; and crucially conscious and unconscious.

Ultimately my contribution to work on malaria and practice is to follow Akram (2013) in drawing attention to the importance of the

---

[13] Haugaard (2008) describes how in place of the word 'habitus', Giddens (1984) uses the term 'practical consciousness', Searle (1995) uses the concept of 'background' and Elias (1994) describes habitus as a kind of 'second nature'.

[14] See Akram (2013) and Akram and Hogan (2015) for a more detailed discussion of the unconscious in Bourdieu's work.

unconscious as it serves to explain the mechanisms that governed why human practice unfolded in the way it did and the effect it had—it was an instrumental part of people's strategic pursuit of power, and built up almost unwittingly over time, as I go on to describe in this book. In other words, the mundane routinisation of social life and the taken-for-granted were fundamental to people's ability to exercise their agency, not just their capacity for explicit reflexivity and conscious intentionality (Akram & Hogan, 2015). This is important because it suggests that practices were orientated towards different goals that were not necessarily straightforwardly, explicitly or even consciously *in response* to malaria, despite the fact malaria was nevertheless implicated in them. As such, strategic practices were at once conscious and unconscious or (un)conscious. This matters because it has implications for how malaria is both conceived of and how it is therefore supposedly 'tackled'. In terms of what people's practice *was* strategically directed towards, namely acquiring power, Dowding (2012) summarises the bewildering plurality in how this fuzzy concept has been conceived of in the social and political sciences, particularly since the twentieth century. Dean (2012) described that early formulations such as that offered by Weber (1978) considered power as '*power-to*'—a probability, capacity, ability or potentiality possessed by an actor (or collective) that enabled them *to* carry out their own will. Others extended this further to claim the endeavour always resulted in '*power-over*' others as a means to achieve this intent whereby those who gained their will did so at the expense of others (Pansardi, 2012). These latter zero-sum conceptions stood in opposition to other more consensual '*power-with*' approaches that located power in a positive-sum game played by collectives of people working together to accomplish aims that could not otherwise be realised in isolation (e.g., Arendt, 1973). These in turn sat in contrast to yet more ideas of power that encompassed both conflictual and consensual elements such as in the work of Foucault (1980) and Giddens (1984). Contention can also be found in the sense that some defined power as obscure and immeasurable (Lukes, 2004), while others claimed it to be measurable and less ambiguous (Dowding, 2019). Some located it in individuals and collectives, others did so in systems and structures (Foucault, 1980). Dowding's (2012) point is that this plurality exists because it reflects the variety of authors' views in which descriptions of power are deployed in line with their own normative commitments and political views about the world. He claims that people used various definitions of power to 'stake out their own territory using a concept that [was] friendly towards their views' (ibid., p. 121). The shapeshifting nature of power is useful to Dowding (2012) because it renders it a theoretical concept that can play different roles in different theories or mechanisms that sought to explain various aspects of human society. As he concluded: 'whilst the definition of "power" matters, it does not matter that much. What is more important is that the term that is adopted in a specific context does the job it is intended to do, and no more' (Dowding, 2012, p. 132). In this regard, I acknowledge that my own use of certain definitions of power fulfils my own theoretical agenda. Specifically, I follow Haugaard (2008) in referring to power as a capacity to take action—a somewhat collaborative endeavour based on our 'ability to impose shared meaning upon things, which gives social actors *power to* do things which they could not otherwise accomplish' (ibid., p. 194). For example, we are able to harness power from the 'natural' world by structuring it according to a system of shared meaning and interacting with others (human and non-human alike) by conceiving of actions as meaningful (ibid.). This basic conception of power as *power to* does not deny that the endeavour can be (and often is) conflictual, oppressive or even violent—that it is *power over* and this certainly comes through in some of the practices described in this book. Rather, it leaves space for other outcomes of power, for other forms to *also* be possible and contained within interactions: 'power can be attributed to structures/systems and agency. It can be dispositional, relational and exercised, ubiquitous, obscure and immeasurable, measurable and visible, consensual and conflictual, zero- and positive-sum, power to, power with and power over, and empowering and dominating' (Vogler, 2016, p. 75). Binaries can thus be reformulated as polarities that attract and repel each other on a continuum but do not necessarily have to exist as mutually exclusive (Dean, 2012).

This more fluid interpretation of power facilitates my intentions to describe people's practices in Bataraza and how they intermingled with malaria. I argue that actors described in this book engaged in (un)conscious strategic practices in their pursuit of achieving various actions in various overlapping fields. As they were enmeshed in complex ecological, political, social, cultural, material and semiotic conditions, their practice was intimately entangled with non-human actors such as malaria and in this way different enactments of the disease were imbricated. This is what I mean when I say malaria *was* (un)conscious strategy—the separation between orientated practice and disease was so ambiguous, it was difficult to disentangle. However, while there was some coordination that allowed various practices (and the malaria that was enacted alongside) to 'hang together' (Mol, 2002), creating consistency and concordance between framings and practices, there was also a level of deviation, contestation and diversion that was not only incorporated or distributed far away enough so as not to cause disruption. In some cases, 'interferences' were actively displaced resulting in incoherence, conflict or even violence as *power over* others was pursued. This was because actors did not exist in one field at a time, their *habitus* was not singular and their strategic pursuits were not isolated. As such, (un)conscious strategies propelled certain versions of malaria forward to be advocated, prioritised and dealt with at the same time as it propelled others to be neglected, side-lined or ignored and *vice versa*. It was this inherent contradiction that explained why malaria, historically and contemporaneously, both frustrated and facilitated life, actions and power acquisition for the Pälawan all at the same time. The role of the anthropologist, in my view, was therefore to describe these contradictions as they took place in context.

Malaria Practices in Palawan

In terms of the specific context, I bring a focus on (un)conscious strategic practice into conversation with a growing body of social scientific research on malaria in the Philippines. According to the WHO (2018a), since 2005, the country reported a 92% reduction in reported malaria cases and 98% reduction in deaths. In 2018, a total of 50 out of 82 provinces were officially declared malaria-free. The remaining cases were mainly of the species *Plasmodium falciparum*[15] and concentrated in what they describe as 'hard-to-reach' areas, mostly on the frontier Island of Palawan. The long, thin island is the largest within the Province of Palawan, itself made up of Palawan Island and a number of smaller surrounding ones (the Calamianes, Balabac Island and the Cuyo Islands) that all lie between the South China Sea and Sulu Sea. Here, the southernmost municipality of Bataraza was identified as an area with particularly high prevalence of malaria. Cases were especially high among forest workers, subsistence farmers and Indigenous Peoples who lived in forested areas (APMEN, 2016). Since seminal works on the links between colonialism and malaria in the Philippines (Anderson, 1992; De Bevoise, 1995), scholarship largely from within the Philippines has more recently drawn attention to the enduring unequal distribution of the disease and access to healthcare among Indigenous People in particular (Bell et al., 2005; Bustos, 2005; Lansang et al., 1997). It has explored local knowledge and treatment patterns in areas such as Agusan del Sur in Mindanao (Miguel et al., 1998, 1999), Bataan in Luzon (Espino & Manderson, 2000; Espino et al., 1997) and Puerto Princesa in Palawan (Castillo-Carandang, 2009) as well as the ways in which this has intersected with healthcare provision. Some have documented the history of malaria control programmes (Asinas, 1992; Espino et al., 2004; Liu et al., 2013) and, more recently, investigated what role community-based health workers have played in shaping patient awareness, access and treatment in Palawan specifically (Angluben et al., 2008; Matsumoto-Takahashi et al., 2013, 2014, 2015, 2018). However, to date, there have been no comprehensive anthropological studies on malaria among the Pälawan or in areas where large numbers of Pälawan live.

At the time of my fieldwork, the Pälawan were officially considered by the Filipino government to be the original inhabitants of Southern Palawan starting from the breach in the mountain range between Quezon and Abo-Abo. It is important to note that, as with all labels, the identity

---

[15] Human malaria is caused by four main different species of *Plasmodium*. The majority of reported cases in the Philippines are due to *P. falciparum*, followed by *P. vivax*; *P. malariae*. Recently, numerous reports have described human malaria caused by a fifth *Plasmodium* species, *Plasmodium knowlesi*, which usually infects macaque monkeys but is now thought to be responsible for less than 1% of cases in the Philippines.

of the Pälawan was somewhat differentiated, fluid and shifting in nature (see Macdonald 2007, pp. 11–16). Describing the historically contingent nature of identity was a feature of much twentieth-century anthropology, to the extent that the assertion that there was variation within any group, permeable boundaries and mixing 'everywhere' was an almost a 'trivial fact' (Eriksen, 2007). Nevertheless, for anthropologists, it remains important to continue to document the specific temporal and spatial contexts in which labels such as 'ethnicity' and 'indigeneity' are created and nego-tiated and ask who articulates their identity in 'Indigenous People' terms, when, why and to what effect (Li, 2000). This is particularly important in light of global Indigenous movements that have taken place since the turn of the twentieth century where idealised portrayals of Indigenous People as stable, unchanged, traditional societies could potentially lead those who do not conform to such stereotypes losing 'credibility' in many arenas (Wawrinec, 2010). As I go on to show in this book, in particular in Chaps. 2 and 4, the categorisation of certain groups in the Philippines as 'Indio[16]' by authorities began during colonisation of the islands by the Spanish in the sixteenth century and continued under the American occupation of the late nineteenth and early twentieth centuries. In par-ticular, as McDermott (2000) suggested, many of the moves by colonial administrations were designed to clear natural resource-rich areas for eco-nomic development or resource extraction, thereby evicting and reset-tling Indigenous Peoples into specific areas, explicitly linking their identity to land (ibid.). More recently, the Indigenous movement in post-colonial Philippines was part of a larger trend which received global insti-tutional support from the United Nations, the World Bank and a host of Non-Governmental Organisations (NGOs) acting across institutional levels (Theriault, 2011). This resulted in the increased official recognition of Indigenous People and their rights by post-authoritarian governments (ibid.). Specifically, the 1987 Philippine Constitution (Article II, Section 22) guaranteed the recognition and promotion of the rights of IPs as state policy. More recently, this was extended through the Indigenous Peoples' Rights Act (IPRA) in 1997. In the same year, the National Commission on Indigenous Peoples (NCIP) was created as the implementing agency

---

[16] Written colonial accounts suggest the Spanish referred to Indigenous People as 'Indio'.

for the IPRA. Since 2008, the NCIP has been under the Department of Environment and Natural Resources (DENR) and was established in order to provide a mechanism for IPs to articulate concerns and address long-standing issues such as ancestral domain claims, thus cementing the link between people and place even further.

The NCIP categorisation and official recognition of IPs in Palawan was evolving but in 2012–2014 when I was there constituted the acknowledgement of the indigeneity of seven other ethnic groups who made up around 20% of the population of the island: the Batak and Tagbanua, who, like the Pälawan, were considered native to the mainland, and the Cuyunon, Agutaynen, Cagayanen, Jama Mapun and Molbog from surrounding islands. However, in reality, boundaries of what constituted 'Pälawan' were more contentious than the NCIP categorisations suggested. Ramil, whom I mentioned at the start of this chapter, was himself ethnically Tagbanua and standing to be a local representative for Indigenous People in Bataraza when I met him. He explained:

Before the NCIP, those eight [ethnic groups] considered themselves [to be] Indigenous to Palawan but not just those—there are even more groups who considered themselves [to be] but they were discounted [by the NCIP]. Some say there are a different group called the Ke'ney. They are like the Pälawan and they live in the trees and are experts in using blow guns. Another group is the Taaw't Batù. They live in the rocks in the mountains but they are not recognised [as a separate group]. The NCIP decided that all of them are just one—the Pälawan. But they speak different languages and have different customs and histories.

As McDermott (2000) pointed out, Indigenous groups, however, have not only been passive subjects of dispossession and state manipulation, as state-recognised and self-defined groups have also used their self-prescribed status to make demands on the state ranging from exclusive access to territories to reparations for past injustices. This has involved forming different alliances such as with media, NGOs and academics. Theriault (2017), Dy (1991) and Macdonald (2007) document how the demonym Palawan has variously been spelled Palaqwan, Pala'wan, 'Palawanän, Pala-wan or Pälawan depending on the dialectical variations within the Palawano language. People I spoke to in Bataraza tended to refer to themselves as Pälawan (where the diacritic indicates the *a* is pronounced as an open back vowel as is in the English 'party'—although often omitted when transcribed into English) and also commonly referred to themselves (and were referred to) as 'natives' or *katutubo* (literally translates as 'innate' in Tagalog) and sometimes 'highlanders', in contrast to 'migrants', 'lowlanders', 'Muslims' or 'Christians'. As described in much more detail throughout the book, in Palawan, 'lowlanders' referred to ethnic groups who settled either temporarily or permanently on this frontier island ranging from Muslim Tausug traders from the Sulu Archipelago (an island chain between the Philippines and the island of Borneo) to Chinese merchants and Christian converts from the Visayas and Luzon in the Philippines (often homogenised and referred to by Pälawan people as '*bisaya*'), particularly following World War II when the government began to offer homesteads on the island to Filipinos from other parts of the country. Across Palawan Island more generally, these distinctions have not however been so clear-cut. A long history of inter-relatedness meant that the vast numbers of conversions to both Islam and Christianity, intermarriage between various groups, heterogeneity of livelihood practices and changing social and political organisation have resulted in ethnic identities that were being produced and reproduced by a variety of structural factors: migration, exchange, government policies, nongovernmental organisations (NGOs), anthropologists and, most crucially perhaps, the peoples of the region themselves (Eder & Fernandez, 1996). In this way, the indigeneity ascribed to and claimed by the Pälawan in some way had 'less to do with blood ties and length of residence and more to do with the group's past and present social position *vis-à-vis* civil society and the state' (Dressler & Turner, 2007, p. 1453). However, as Smith (2020) describes, in Bataraza specifically, there was a sharper topographical and ethnic relief between Indigenous, state-owned uplands and migrant, privately titled lowlands that made this municipality stand apart from others on the island to some extent as it felt somewhat more 'sealed off' from the its neighbours. Practically, this was due to the Mantalingahan mountain range which cuts through Bataraza, separating it from the territory to the west and north to some extent, but within the municipality itself, there was a palpable absence of both governmental, NGOs and

Civil Society Organisations (CSOs) especially around environmental protection in the uplands where many Pälawan reside, unlike the rest of the island. As such, communities in higher elevations in particular seemed to live in relative separation from state infrastructure and 'lowlander' life (ibid.) only really venturing into the main town for *arawan* (Tagalog for wage labour) to access health services and to sell produce in the market. In turn, migrants that I knew seldom traversed the terrain to Pälawan communities and were rather shocked that a single woman like myself dared to do so, fearing I would be poisoned, subject to 'tap-tap' (a curse brought on by being tapped on the shoulder) or kidnapped by Islamic separatists thought to 'hide out' in the forests of Bataraza.

Although the Pälawan I worked with predominantly used Palawano, part of the Meso-Philippine group of languages (a branch of the Austronesian language family), a combination of the rise in migration, religious conversion and the growth in government education meant that an increasing number also used the national language of Tagalog as well as English, especially younger people. While many of my interactions with professionals, health staff or migrant settlers took place in English or Tagalog, I relied heavily on one of my principal gatekeepers, Ramil (whom I discuss in more detail below), to translate Palawano for me as well as other dialects used by non-Pälawan groups, especially in the early months while my language proficiency improved. Throughout the book, translations of important Palawano terms are provided and I indicate where participants specifically used Tagalog or English words in ways that seemed relevant. Many Pälawan employed a number of rhetorical devices and strategies in order to think, discuss, deliberate and decide, make judgements and resolve conflict (Dy, 1991). This was especially the case when talking to older community members and in particular Chieftains or *panglimas* (Pälawan leaders) who would sometimes answer questions in the form of riddles or proverbs. In these situations, I depended on the knowledge and experience of Ramil to decode and transpose subtle meanings and respond in appropriate ways that remained elusive to me.

The data presented in this book were collected between April 2012 and February 2014, as part of my doctoral thesis in medical anthropology. As stated above, my interest lay in documenting the practices of many actors in Bataraza in a broad sense but in particular in relation to malaria and its intersection with life for the Pälawan. In order to attend to practices, engaging in ethnographic methods was vital as it allowed me to directly participate in and observe the 'activities, events, buildings, instruments, procedures, and so on' (Mol, 2002, p. 32) that were crucial to how practice was enacted through space and time. For Bueger (2014), the core elements of practice were 'implicit knowledge [and] bodily movements' (ibid., p. 388) that could be accessed in participant observation, but as Haugaard (2008) noted, focussing on *habitus* also involves attending to language and the way in which actors 'distance themselves from their *habitus* by making it discursive. In this process, they become "strangers" to themselves. The capacity for reflexive description contains within it the possibility for the redescription of reality as something else. *Habitus* ... can be consciously changed through being made discursive' (ibid., p. 193). Talking to people, both informally by nature of living in Bataraza and through more formal in-depth interviews, allowed me to attend to not only unconscious (bodily) elements of practice gained through participant observation but also to conscious (discursive) elements and the ways in which the two related.

Specifically, for 13 months I lived in the only licenced pharmacy located in Marangas, the Centre of Bataraza, with Illaine, her family and her three staff. Day-to-day life for me involved observing patient/provider practices as they unfolded alongside family life—playing with the children, preparing and eating food, practising Tagalog or just idly perching on a stool watching life (and the ever-changing weather) unfurl. The wooden pharmacy, built by Illaine and her late husband, was located in the centre of the *poblacion* (town centre), and its large open front faced out onto hills and mountains in the background and the town square in the foreground, where people congregated to go to the bank or municipal government, shopped in the market, crowded round TVs watching sport (including the London Olympics at that time) or simply chatted whilst waiting for their phones to charge using the pharmacy's generator (being one of the few homes in the town to have such a luxury). Its central location afforded me access to multiple 'fields' where public practice unfolded such as in local government meetings, town festivals, sporting events, cultural and artistic performances and much more mundane, everyday social interactions but this 'town life' was dominated by the migrants of

Bataraza who lived in lower elevations of the municipality. Crucially, the Rural Health Unit (RHU) was just a stone's throw away and through this proximity I gained insight into the 'formal' healthcare sector and how people from the Pälawan community accessed and interacted with services beyond the pharmacy. The Medical Technician and Coordinator of Vector-Borne Diseases, Danny, was the first person I met in Bataraza and guided me throughout my stay. Through him, I was able to spend a lot of time in the RHU and assisted health staff in some of the practices that they conducted on 'medical missions' where they screened for malaria, distributed mosquito nets and disseminated educational information. I accompanied Danny, *Barangay* Health Workers, Rapid Diagnostic Test technicians and the malaria Community Relations Officer on their rounds in Pälawan communities and, as such, was able to directly observe, and in some cases participate in, practices.

My work was largely concentrated around the *poblacion* and closely surrounding areas. Bataraza is subdivided into 22 *barangays*, the smallest administrative division in the Philippines. Initially guided by Danny and Ramil, I was able to meet many people from Pälawan communities in *barangays* where both men had lived and worked over many years. Their positions were somewhat unique. Danny, for example, although from Manila, had lived in Bataraza for almost a decade and given his prominent role in the community was almost like a celebrity. He seemed to know everyone and everyone to know him. In some ways it was not surprising given the RHU (and extended posts) was the main site responsible for providing formal healthcare to its 64,000 or so inhabitants. As well as his dedicated work in health which took him to all corners of the municipality, Danny had also lived more intensively with upland communities as part of his involvement in the Palawan Tropical Forest Protection Program (that ran between 1995 and 2002 and is described in more detail in Chap. 4). Through him, I was able to gain access to areas where malaria was most prevalent according to RHU records and in particular meet people from Pälawan communities with expertise in health such as the professionals I describe in Chap. 5 as well as those involved in conservation and issues related to land that I describe in Chap. 4. Ramil, himself ethnically Tagbanua, had moved to Bataraza in 2004 as pastor of a small Pentecostal church belonging to the Assemblies of God Fellowship.

Initially, and perhaps naturally, the people that he introduced me to were from his congregation (i.e., ethnic Pälawans who had converted to Christianity). However, as time went on, he was also able to introduce me to a much wider array of individuals and communities. In addition to being a pastor, both he and his wife worked as community teachers for IP groups through the Alternative Learning System (ALS)—an informal education system that facilitated out-of-school pupils to study towards qualifying exams—and Ramil himself was standing to be an IP representative in Bataraza. His wife, Babydan, also Tagbanua, was a *Barangay* Health Worker and as such well-established in Pälawan communities too. Both were from a bloodline of *babalyans* (Tagbanua healers) and therefore possessed a great deal of knowledge relating to Pälawan healing practices (as there were many similarities) but crucially were known and respected by many healers whose practices were somewhat esoteric and purposively kept private, especially from outsiders. Ramil's unique social position in Bataraza was coupled with his fluency in dialects such as Tagbanwa, Palawano and Ilocano (as well as Tagalog and English). Consequently, he had experience translating for three or four other foreign researchers, including anthropologists. This made him well-versed in anthropological research approaches (especially the notion of engaging in lots of *chika-chika* or chit chat to build rapport) and ideas, and was attentive to translation and language in a way that an anthropologist can only dream of when having to confront their own linguistic inadequacies. Consequently, Ramil and Babydan worked in a wide variety of areas and were well-known and trusted by many members of the Pälawan community for a host of reasons beyond their association with the church.

Danny and Ramil's relationship with the Pälawan people that I met, local expertise and overall competencies were invaluable as health staff and missionaries were among the few 'migrant' groups who seemed to venture into the uplands and mix with Indigenous communities. As intimated above, 'in contrast to the fluidity that characterise[d] identity politics in other areas of the island, the ethnic boundaries between indigenous peoples and Filipinos of migrant settler origin [were] relatively less malleable' (Smith, 2020, p. 27) in Bataraza. The access they were able to broker on my behalf was even more significant due to the heavy restrictions imposed on me by local oversight agencies, mainly the NCIP (as I describe in much more detail in Chap. 4). Due to restrictions imposed by them I was not able to live on Pälawan ancestral lands with Pälawan people and so my encounters were largely through spending days participating in more formal activities such as those run by the RHU, ALSs or the church, conducting interviews, observing and generally 'hanging out' as people carried on with everyday life in their homes, gardens, farms of community halls. I was invited to weddings, funerals, community meetings and religious ceremonies, and to take part in everything from collecting medicinal plants and farming to constructing and moving houses. A significant part of my doctoral work also involved conducting an intensive Participatory-Action-Research (PAR) project related to malaria with children in elementary schools. I document my use of photovoice in much more detail in various publications (Black et al., 2018; Iskander, 2015a, b, 2019) and return to it in the Conclusion of this book in terms of the implications it had for (un)conscious practice and health-related interventions. However, the relevance for this methodological account is that I spent a considerable amount of time in schools with predominantly Pälawan children who pictorially documented their lives, practices and what malaria meant to them over 15 weeks, producing literally hundreds of photographs, narratives and outputs (such as exhibitions, posters, a film and a series of community events). These data, alongside over 3000 photographs and audio recordings that I took as well as diagrams, drawings and maps, meant I had wide-ranging access to non-textual descriptions of practice. 'Being there' (Borneman & Hammoudi, 2009) meant that although I could not subject *myself* to all of the contingencies that play upon the lives of the people I met in Bataraza, most notably the Pälawan, I was able to gain a small window of insight into different kinds of practices, their dual (un)conscious nature, the way malaria was implicated along the way and, ultimately, the way power emerged through interactions and was shaped alongside them.

Malaria as (Un)conscious Strategy

Throughout this book, I use the English term malaria to denote the bio-medical term that implies a specific aetiology, presentation and treatment in line with this medical system. For some participants, mainly health staff working in 'formal' healthcare settings (hospitals, clinics, etc.) as well as some government leaders, this was what they meant when they used the term. In contrast, I use the Tagalog translation *malarya* to echo other participants' conception of a similar but broader illness category as I go on to describe. There was of course overlap and the terms were somewhat interchangeable. In order to illustrate my arguments, the book is structured in the following way: in Chap. 2, I describe the ways in which fever and malaria were implicated in various historical (un)conscious practices orientated towards achieving dominance and oppression. Largely based on an analysis of secondary sources, I describe some of the significant ecological, economic, political, social and cultural changes that took place in the Philippines during the colonial exploitation of the islands particularly by the Spanish and Americans during the sixteenth to early twentieth centuries. When the first Spanish explorers arrived in the mid-sixteenth century, *paludismo* (marsh fever), considered by the colonisers to emanate from the foreign landscape, initially offered some protection to small clusters of Indigenous People residing in the forested uplands who were either ignored or actively avoided by the administration. However, as Spanish economic interests changed and they embarked on turning the islands into producer and exporter of agriculture commodities in order to maintain control over their colonies, they transformed the landscape across the archipelago, eventually leading to *paludismo* being the biggest killer of Indigenous populations and colonisers alike across the islands by the end of the nineteenth century. While this threat to life and livelihood may well have played a part in spurring popular resistance movements against the Spanish, as revolutionaries sought to seize control, it appears fever was more directly associated with a new colonial power's attempts to oppress the island and its inhabitants yet again. Under American occupation, malaria as it was now called was implicated in scientifically and biomedically grounded attempts to tame the supposed savagery of the natural world and the foreign bodies that inhabited it. By situating the history of malaria in the context of these practices, the effects of which linger into the present day, I demonstrate how malaria lost and gained power due its entanglement with human relations enacted in, around and out of its name. Malaria was therefore advertently and inadvertently enmeshed in various groups' efforts to secure different kinds of economic, political and social control of the islands in the field of colonial encounters.

Chapter 3 focuses more explicitly on the twentieth- and twenty-first-century post-colonial context to set the scene for the way in which malaria was implicated in various contemporary actors' (un)conscious practices orientated towards achieving what they described as different kinds of 'progress'. Specifically, I move to my own ethnographic findings and describe how malaria was conceived of and dealt with by current health workers employed in implementing health policy in Bataraza in 2012–2014. I show how, as global medical citizens, they were caught between responsibilities to the post-colonial nation state and a transnational network of organisations that also governed the nature of, access to and inclusion within healthcare for the citizens of Bataraza. By focussing on how the three main staff responsible for designing and delivering malaria-related initiatives (the Municipal Health Officer, the Medical Health Technician and the Community Relation Officer) framed and handled malaria in the field of official malaria control programmes, I describe how certain conceptions and practices tended to be appropriated over others alongside these actors' goals of achieving different kinds of 'progress' for both themselves and the communities they served. The resultant 'malaria of progress' as I call it was cast as a 'top priority' and co-opted into wider projects of 'curing', 'educating' and ultimately 'empowering' the Pälawan people whom it affected most as well as these actors' efforts to 'dutifully' meet their obligations to the transnational state in reaching targets and securing momentum and investment around health service delivery. As they pushed forward with enacting this malaria of progress, these actors deprioritised the malaria that was less of a concern to most Pälawan people, the more urgent health and social issues that they faced, and in turn the practices and knowledge that they possessed to enable them to live better lives.

In Chap. 4 I describe the global, national and regional landscape of conservation and Indigenous rights and show how this was linked to the way in which malaria was implicated in various other actors' (un)conscious practices that were orientated towards achieving 'sustainable development'. I describe how malaria was conceived of and dealt with by locally based government officials in Bataraza who discursively and practically aligned with similar agendas. In the field of local governance, actors such as the Mayor and some *Barangay* Captains and NCIP-validated 'Chieftains' of Pälawan communities framed and dealt with malaria as though it was a thing of the 'past', eliminated due to their success at pushing forth with economic and social development. The 'malaria of development' was co-opted into these leaders' efforts to win votes, retain political office and boost economic profit through promoting activities such as agricultural development, tourism and mining on ancestral lands. By lauding an eliminated malaria as a success story of development, these actors simultaneously fuelled and silenced the presence of an emerging and persistent malaria that conversely flourished out of the changing landscape. The malaria that endured as a problem for Pälawan people was however drawn into their own resistance efforts to retain power over their ancestral lands and livelihoods.

Chapter 5 focuses on the therapeutic landscape of Bataraza where multiple healing possibilities were available, experienced and understood. As such, malaria/*malarya* was intertwined with various actors' practices that were orientated towards establishing themselves as legitimate 'professionals' in contrast to the lay population. Accordingly, I describe how it was conceived of and dealt with by four healers: a Pälawan *balayan* (healer); a *manghihilot* (bone setter); a *Barangay* health worker; and a pharmacist who had all undergone extensive training in the field of healing following a 'calling' into their respective professions. The esoteric knowledge and practices that they acquired gave them all access to a power that their patients did not possess—the ability to 'see' the 'unseen' circumstances that resulted in sickness, which they diagnosed and healed in the acute phases of illness using various bodily techniques and potent but ambiguous objects. As a result, the 'hidden' 'malaria/*malarya* of professionalisation' was co-opted into their (un)conscious strategies orientated towards achieving legitimisation and control in a therapeutic landscape where many competing treatment options existed. The sickness that was 'uncovered' and dealt with was to some degree at the expense of lay expertise and the kinds of malaria that non-professional Pälawan people contended with every day, over a lifetime and without the use of recognised professionals, esoteric knowledge and specialist tools.

In Chap. 6 I turn my attention to a final group of strategic practices that I argue were (un)consciously orientated towards achieving a kind of equilibrium as a means for people to deal with and fend off sickness and misfortune that made them feel *sakit* (Tagalog for pain or sickness). I describe how a broad category of what is referred to as *malarya* in Tagalog was conceived of and dealt with by people engaged in everyday struggles to prevent (through the avoidance of disequilibrium) and heal (through restoring equilibrium) it as a means to handle the acute and chronic nature of the disease (Castillo-Carandang, 2009) over a lifetime. By giving examples of how three people from the Pälawan community, Narcita, Isabelle and Bernas, worked towards maintaining balance within their bodies, social relations and the wider cosmos, I show how certain conceptions and practices of *malarya* were appropriated over others alongside these actors' rhetoric and practice of 'equilibrium'. The *malarya* that was enacted as a result was felt as an intra- and extra-bodily state and implicated in attempts to carefully weigh the body's interaction with the external environment or intrusive agents; maintain harmonious social relations and emotional lives; and to restore cosmological balance by appeasing or honouring relations between humans and the non-human world. As they pushed forward with these acts of 'ethical choreography' (Stonington, 2020), these Pälawan people, like many others, consulted and interacted with a range of human and non-human actors, far beyond the health leaders, local government actors and professionals described thus far in order to assemble 'good' ways to live.

Finally, in the Conclusion, I summarise what I learnt from the experiences that were shared with me and discuss the implications for approaching malaria in this context and beyond.

References

Abimbola, S., & Pai, M. (2020). Will global health survive its decolonisation? *The Lancet (British edition), 396*(10263), 1627–1628.

Ajzen, I., & Fishbein, M. (1973). Attitudinal and normative variables as predictors of specific behavior. *Journal of Personality and Social Psychology, 27*, 41–57.

Akram, S. (2013). Fully unconscious and prone to habit: The characteristics of agency in the structure and agency dialectic. *Journal for the Theory of Social Behaviour, 43*(1), 45–65.

Akram, S., & Hogan, A. (2015). On reflexivity and the conduct of the self in everyday life: Reflections on Bourdieu and Archer: On reflexivity and the conduct of the self in everyday life. *The British Journal of Sociology, 66*(4), 605–625.

Anderson, W. (1992). Where every prospect pleases and only man is vile: Laboratory medicine as colonial discourse. *Critical inquiry, 18*(3), 506–529.

Anderson, W. (2004). Natural histories of infectious disease: Ecological vision in twentieth-century biomedical science. *Osiris (Bruges), 19*, 39–61.

Angluben, R. U., Trudeau, M. R., Kano, S., & Tongol-Rivera, P. (2008). Kilusan Ligtas Malaria: Advancing social mobilization towards sustainable malaria control in the province of Palawan, the Philippines. *Tropical Medicine and Health, 36*(1), 45–49.

APMEN. (2016). *Asia Pacific Malaria Elimination Network Country briefing: Eliminating malaria in the Philippines.* https://www.aplma.org/apmen/apmen/Resources/Country%20Briefings/Philippines2016_Final.pdf

Arendt, H. (1973). *The origins of totalitarianism* (Vol. 244). Houghton Mifflin Harcourt.

Asinas, C. Y. (1992). Current status of malaria and control activities in the Philippines. *Southeast Asian Journal of Tropical Medicine and Public Health, 23*(Suppl 4), 55–59.

Batista, E. P., Costa, E. F., & Silva, A. A. (2014). Anopheles darlingi (Diptera: Culicidae) displays increased attractiveness to infected individuals with *Plasmodium vivax* gametocytes. *Parasites and Vectors, 7*, 251.

Beisel, U. (2010). *Who bites back first?: Malaria control in Ghana and the politics of co-existence.* ProQuest Dissertations Publishing.

Beisel, U. (2015). Markets and mutations: Mosquito nets and the politics of disentanglement in global health. *Geoforum, 66*, 146–155.

Bell, D., Go, R., Miguel, C., Parks, W., & Bryan, J. (2005). Unequal treatment access and malaria risk in a community-based intervention program in the Philippines. *Southeast Asian Journal of Tropical Medicine and Public Health, 36*(3), 578–586.

Black, G. F., Davies, A., Iskander, D., & Chambers, M. (2018). Reflections on the ethics of participatory visual methods to engage communities in global health research. *Problemi di bioetica, 29*(1), 22–38.

Borneman, J., & Hammoudi, A. (Eds.). (2009). *Being there: The fieldwork encounter and the making of truth.* University of California Press.

Bourdieu, P. (1977). *Outline of a theory of practice.* Cambridge University Press.

Bourdieu, P. (1990). *The logic of practice*. Stanford University Press.
Bourdieu, P., & Wacquant, L. J. (1992). *An invitation to reflexive sociology*. University of Chicago Press.
Brown, H., & Kelly, A. H. (2014). Material proximities and hotspots: Toward an anthropology of viral hemorrhagic fevers. *Medical Anthropology Quarterly, 28*(2), 280–303.
Bueger, C. (2014). Pathways to practice: Praxiography and international politics. *European Political Science Review, 6*(03), 383–406.
Bustos, M. D. G. (2005). The pharmacokinetics and pharmacodynamics of anti-malarials: A new approach in the treatment of malaria: The Philippine experience. *International Journal of Antimicrobial Agents, 26*, S38–S38.
Busula, A. O., Bousema, T., Mweresa, C. K., Masiga, D., Logan, J. G., Sauerwein, R. W., … de Boer, J. G. (2017). Gametocytemia and attractiveness of *Plasmodium falciparum*-infected Kenyan children to Anopheles gambiae mosquitoes. *The Journal of Infectious Diseases, 216*(3), 291–295.
Castillo-Carandang, N. T. (2009). Notions of risk and vulnerability to malaria. *Acta Medica Philippina, 43*(3), 48–55.
Cator, L. J., Lynch, P. A., Thomas, M. B., & Read, A. F. (2014). Alterations in mosquito behaviour by malaria parasites: Potential impact on force of infection. *Malaria Journal, 13*(1), 164.
Chandler, C., & Beisel, U. (2017). The anthropology of malaria: Locating the social. *Medical Anthropology, 36*(5), 411–421.
Chandler, C., Mangham, L., Njei, A. N., Achonduh, O., Mbacham, W. F., & Wiseman, V. (2012). 'As a clinician, you are not managing lab results, you are managing the patient': How the enactment of malaria at health facilities in Cameroon compares with new WHO guidelines for the use of malaria tests. *Social Science & Medicine, 74*.
Cohn, S. (2014). From health behaviours to health practices: An introduction. *Sociology of Health & Illness, 36*(2), 157–162.
Cox, F. E. G. (2010). History of the discovery of the malaria parasites and their vectors. *Parasites & Vectors, 3*(1), 5.
Crossley, N. (2001). The phenomenological habitus and its construction. *Theory and Society, 30*(1), 81–120. http://www.jstor.org/stable/658063
De Bevoise, K. (1995). *Agents of apocalypse: epidemic disease in the colonial Philippines*. Princeton, N.J.; Chichester: Princeton University Press.
Dean, M. (2012). The signature of power. *Journal of Political Power, 5*(1), 101–117. https://doi.org/10.1080/2158379X.2012.659864
Dowding, K. (2012). Why should we care about the definition of power? *Journal of Political Power, 5*(1), 119–135. https://doi.org/10.1080/2158379X.2012.661917

Dowding, K. (2019). *Rational choice and political power*. Policy Press.

Dressler, W., & Turner, S. (2007). The persistence of social differentiation in the Philippine uplands. *Journal of Development Studies, 44*(10), 450–1473.

Dy, D. (1991). *'Preserving Palawan', Bountiful Palawan*. Aurora Publications.

Eckl, J. (2017). The social lives of global policies against malaria: Conceptual considerations, past experiences, and current issues. *Medical Anthropology, 36*(5), 422–435. https://doi.org/10.1080/01459740.2017.1315667

Eder, J. F., & Fernandez, J. (1996). *Palawan at the crossroads: Development and environment on a Philippine frontier*. Ateneo de Manila University Press.

Elias, N. (1994). *The civilizing process: The development of manners*. Blackwell.

Eriksen, T. H. (2007). Creolization in anthropological theory and in Mauritius. In C. Stewart (Ed.), *Creolization: His-tory, ethnography, theory* (pp. 153–177). Left Coast Press.

Espino, F., & Manderson, L. (2000). Treatment seeking for malaria in Morong, Bataan, the Philippines. *Social Science & Medicine, 50*(9), 1309–1316. https://doi.org/10.1016/s0277-9536(99)00379-2

Espino, F., Manderson, L., Acuin, C., Domingo, F., & Ventura, E. (1997). Perceptions of malaria in a low endemic area in the Philippines: Transmission and prevention of disease. *Acta Tropica, 63*(4), 221–239. http://www.science-direct.com/science/article/pii/S0001706X96006237

Espino, F., Beltran, M., & Carisma, B. (2004). Malaria control through municipalities in the Philippines: Struggling with the mandate of decentralized health programme management. *International Journal of Health Planning and Management, 19*, S155–S166. https://doi.org/10.1002/hpm.782

Foucault, M. (1980). *Power/knowledge: Selected interviews and other writings, 1972–1977*. Vintage.

Giddens, A. (1984). *The constitution of society*. Polity Press.

Govella, N. J., Chaki, P. P., & Killeen, G. F. (2013). Entomological surveillance of behavioural resilience and resistance in residual malaria vector populations. *Malaria Journal, 12*(1), 124. https://doi.org/10.1186/1475-2875-12-124

Haraway, D. J. (2008). *When species meet*. University of Minnesota Press.

Haugaard, M. (2008). Power and habitus. *Journal of Power, 1*(2), 189–206. https://doi.org/10.1080/17540290802227593

Heidegger, M., 1967. *Being and time*. Oxford: Blackwell.

Hochbaum, G. M. (1956). Why people seek diagnostic X-rays. *Public Health Reports, 71*, 377–380.

Hoffman, M. A. (2016). *Malaria, mosquitoes, and maps: Practices and articulations of malaria control in British India and WWII*. eScholarship, University of California.

Hsu, E. (2006a). The history of qing hao in the Chinese materia medica. *Transactions of the Royal Society of Tropical Medicine and Hygiene, 100*(6), 505–508. https://doi.org/10.1016/j.trstmh.2005.09.020

Hsu, E. (2006b). Reflections on the 'discovery' of the antimalarial qinghao. *British Journal of Clinical Pharmacology, 61*(6), 666–670. https://doi.org/10.1111/j.1365-2125.2006.02673.x

Iskander, D. (2015a). Parasites, power, and photography. *Trends in Parasitology, 32*(1), 2–3.

Iskander, D. (2015b). Re-imaging malaria in the Philippines: How photovoice can help to re-imagine malaria. *Malaria Journal, 14*(1), 257.

Iskander, D. (2019). How photographs 'empower' bodies to act differently. In A. Parkhusrt & T. Carroll (Eds.), *Medical materialities: Toward a material culture of medical anthropology* (1st ed.). Routledge.

Kelly, A. H., & Beisel, U. (2011). Neglected malarias: The frontlines and back alleys of global health. *BioSocieties, 6*(1), 71–87. https://doi.org/10.1057/biosoc.2010.42

Kirksey, S. E., & Helmreich, S. (2010). The emergence of multispecies ethnography. *Cultural Anthropology, 25*(4), 545–576. https://doi.org/10.1111/j.1548-1360.2010.01069.x

Lacroix, R., Mukabana, W. R., Gouagna, L. C., & Koella, J. C. (2005). Malaria infection increases attractiveness of humans to mosquitoes. *PLoS Biology, 3*(9), e298. https://doi.org/10.1371/journal.pbio.0030298

Langwick, S. A. (2007). Devils, parasites, and fierce needles: Healing and the politics of translation in Southern Tanzania. *Science, Technology & Human Values, 32*(1), 88–117. https://doi.org/10.1177/0162243906293887

Lansang, M. A., Belizario, V. Y., Bustos, M. D., Saul, A., & Aguirre, A. (1997). Risk factors for infection with malaria in a low endemic community in Bataan, the Philippines. *Acta Tropica, 63*(4), 257–265. https://doi.org/10.1016/S0001-706X(96)00625-0

Latour, B. (1988). *The pasteurization of France / Bruno Latour* (A. Sheridan & J. Law, Trans.). Harvard University Press.

Law, J. (2008). Actor network theory and material semiotics. In B. S. Turner (Ed.), *The new Blackwell companion to social theory* (pp. 141–158). Wiley-Blackwell.

Li, T. M. (2000). Articulating indigenous identity in Indonesia: Resource politics and the tribal slot. *Comparative Studies in Society and History, 42*(1), 149–179. https://doi.org/10.1017/S0010417500002632

Lindsay, S., Kirby, M., Baris, E., & Bos, R. (2004). *Environmental management for malaria control in the East Asia and Pacific (EAP) region*. World Bank.

Liu, J. X., Newby, G., Brackery, A., Smith Gueye, C., Candari, C. J., Escubil, L. R., … Baquilod, M. (2013). Determinants of malaria program expenditures during elimination: Case study evidence from select provinces in the Philippines. *PLoS ONE, 8*(9).

Lukes, S. (2004). *Power: A radical view.* Macmillan International Higher Education.

Macdonald, C., J-H. (2007). Uncultural behavior, an anthropological investigation of suicide in the southern Philippines. Honolulu: University of Hawai'i Press.

Marsland, R. (2007). The modern traditional healer: Locating "hybridity" in modern traditional medicine, Southern Tanzania. *Journal of Southern African Studies, 33*(4), 751–765.

Matsumoto-Takahashi, E. L., Tongol-Rivera, P., Villacorte, E. A., Angluben, R. U., Yasuoka, J., Kano, S., & Jimba, M. (2013). Determining the active role of microscopists in community awareness-raising activities for malaria prevention: A cross-sectional study in Palawan, the Philippines. *Malaria Journal, 12*, 384. https://doi.org/10.1186/1475-2875-12-384

Matsumoto-Takahashi, E. L. A., Tongol-Rivera, P., Villacorte, E. A., Angluben, R. U., Yasuoka, J., Kano, S., & Jimba, M. (2014). Determining the impact of community awareness-raising activities on the prevention of malaria transmission in Palawan, the Philippines. *Parasitology International, 63*(3), 519–526. https://doi.org/10.1016/j.parint.2014.01.008

Matsumoto-Takahashi, E. L. A., Tongol-Rivera, P., Villacorte, E. A., Angluben, R. U., Jimba, M., & Kano, S. (2015). Patient knowledge on malaria symptoms is a key to promoting universal access of patients to effective malaria treatment in Palawan, the Philippines. *PLOS ONE, 10*(6), e0127858. https://doi.org/10.1371/journal.pone.0127858

Matsumoto-Takahashi, E. L. A., Tongol-Rivera, P., Villacorte, E. A., Angluben, R. U., Jimba, M., & Kano, S. (2018). Bottom-up approach to strengthen community-based malaria control strategy from community health workers' perceptions of their past, present, and future: A qualitative study in Palawan, Philippines. *Tropical Medicine and Health, 46*, 24–24. https://doi.org/10.1186/s41182-018-0105-x

McDermott, M. H. (2000). *Boundaries and pathways: Indigenous identity, ancestral domain, and forest use in Palawan, the Philippines.* Rutgers University.

Michie, S., Johnston, M., Abraham, C., Lawton, R., Parker, D., & Walker, A. (2005). Making psychological theory useful for implementing evidence based practice: A consensus approach. *Quality and Safety in Health Care, 14*(1), 26–33. https://doi.org/10.1136/qshc.2004.011155

Miguel, C. A., Manderson, L., & Lansang, M. A. (1998). Patterns of treatment for malaria in Tayabas, The Philippines: Implications for control. *Tropical Medicine & International Health, 3*(5), 413–421. http://www.ncbi.nlm.nih. gov/entrez/query.fcgi?cmd=Retrieve&db=PubMed&dopt=Citation& list_uids=9623948

Miguel, C. A., Tallo, V. L., Manderson, L., & Lansang, M. A. (1999). Local knowledge and treatment of malaria in Agusan del Sur, the Philippines. *Social Science & Medicine, 48*(5), 607–618. https://doi.org/10.1016/ s0277-9536(98)00352-9

Mitchell, T. (2002). *Rule of experts: Egypt, techno-politics, modernity.* University of California Press.

Mol, A. (2002). *The body multiple: Ontology in medical practice.* Duke University Press.

Nading, A. M. (2014). *Mosquito trails: Ecology, health and the politics of entanglement.* University of California Press.

Okumu, F. (2020). The fabric of life: What if mosquito nets were durable and widely available but insecticide-free? *Malaria Journal, 19*(1).

Packard, R. M. (2014). The origins of antimalarial-drug resistance. *New England Journal of Medicine, 371*(5), 397–399. https://doi.org/10.1056/ NEJMp1403340

Pansardi, P. (2012). Power to and power over: Two distinct concepts of power? *Journal of Political Power, 5*(1), 73–89. https://doi.org/10.108 0/2158379x.2012.658278

Parker, M., & Allen, T. (2014). De-politicizing parasites: Reflections on attempts to control the control of neglected tropical diseases. *Medical Anthropology: Cross-Cultural Studies in Health and Illness, 33*(3), 223–239.

Popovici, J., Roesch, C., & Rougeron, V. (2020). The enigmatic mechanisms by which *Plasmodium vivax* infects Duffy-negative individuals. *PLOS Pathogens, 16*(2), e1008258.

Roy, R. D. (2017). *Malarial subjects: Empire, medicine and nonhumans in British India, 1820–1909.* Cambridge University Press.

Searle, J. (1995). *The construction of social reality.* Penguin.

Smith, W. (2020). *Mountains of blame climate and culpability in the Philippine Uplands / Will Smith.* Seattle University of Washington Press.

Stonington, S. D. (2020). Karma masters: The ethical wound, hauntological choreography, and complex personhood in Thailand. *American Anthropologist, 122*(4), 759–770.

Sweetman, P. (2003). Twenty-first century dis-ease? Habitual reflexivity or the reflexive habitus. *The Sociological Review (Keele), 51*(4), 526.

Theriault, N. (2011). The micropolitics of indigenous environmental movements in the Philippines. *Development and Change, 42*(6), 1417–1440.

Theriault, N. (2017). A forest of dreams: Ontological multiplicity and the fantasies of environmental government in the Philippines. *Political Geography, 58*, 114–127. https://doi.org/10.1016/j.polgeo.2015.09.004

Tsing, A. (2012). Unruly edges: Mushrooms as companion species: For Donna Haraway. *Environmental Humanities, 1*(1), 141–154. https://doi.org/10.121 5/22011919-3610012

Veenstra, G., & Burnett, P. J. (2014). A relational approach to health practices: Towards transcending the agency-structure divide. *Sociology of Health & Illness, 36*(2), 187–198. https://doi.org/10.1111/1467-9566.12105

Vogler, G. (2016). Power between habitus and reflexivity – Introducing Margaret Archer to the power debate. *Journal of Political Power, 9*(1), 65–82. https://doi.org/10.1080/2158379X.2016.1149309

Wawrinec, C. (2010). Tribality and indigeneity in Malaysia and Indonesia. *The Stanford Journal of East Asian Affairs, 10*(1).

Weber, M. (1978). *Economy and society: An outline of interpretive sociology.* University of California Press.

Wekesa, J. W., Copeland, R. S., & Mwangi, R. W. (1992). Effect of *Plasmodium falciparum* on blood feeding behavior of naturally infected Anopheles mosquitoes in Western Kenya. *The American Journal of Tropical Medicine and Hygiene, 47*(4), 484–488. https://doi.org/10.4269/ajtmh.1992.47.484

World Health Organization. (2018a). *Eliminating malaria with better monitoring in the Philippines.* https://www.who.int/westernpacific/news/feature-stories/detail/eliminating-malaria-with-better-monitoring-in-the-philippines

World Health Organization. (2018b). *Global report on insecticide resistance in malaria vectors: 2010–2016.* https://www.who.int/malaria/publications/atoz/9789241514057/en/

World Health Organization. (2020a). *Malaria fact sheet.* https://www.who.int/news-room/fact-sheets/detail/malaria

World Health Organization. (2020b). *World malaria report 2020: 20 years of global progress and challenges.* https://www.who.int/teams/global-malaria-programme/reports/world-malaria-report-2020

2

Practices of Oppression

Introduction

> One realizes his insignificance before the grandeur of Nature that sur-
> rounds him, and afraid of having surprised its secrets, there surges an irre-
> sistible impulse to abandon such dark and mysterious places. (*Extract from
> Ramon Jordana y Morera's report for the Universal Exposition in
> Philadelphia, 1876*[1])

The dark and mysterious places that Jordana, Inspector General of mountains, forests and lands for the colonial Inspección de Montes, felt compelled to abandon were the foothills that were common to many areas of
the Philippines. For early Spanish invaders, these belts of land between
plain and mountain were to be avoided, teeming with *paludismo* (meaning marsh in Spanish, derived from Latin *palus*) or what the Italians called
'*mal' aria*' (bad air), supposed foetid emanations from the squalid mists
and miasmas of the decomposing vegetation, where small clusters of

---

[1] Cited in De Bevoise (1995, p. 142).

'*Indios*'[2]—as they were referred to—lived. The trajectory of malaria parasites in the Philippines is intimately linked to this forest ecology as the primary mosquitoes that carry them in this region, *A. minimus flavirostris*, thrive in higher altitudes (800–2000 feet) and the shady, cool, wet environments that the trees and streams afford. However, for early Spanish colonisers, this link between the raging fever and mosquitoes was not well established. As such, the 'dark and mysterious' forests offered some limited initial protection from colonial encroachment to the Indigenous People that lived or retreated there—among whom outbreaks of disease, although likely deadly when they did occur, were rarely experienced and remained relatively contained (Newson, 1999). However, by the end of the nineteenth century the situation was altogether different, and the roots of the problem can be traced back through the 350-year colonial occupation that began in 1521. Although Spanish interference was initially confined to the lowlands, by the late nineteenth century their economic interests had changed, leading to the mass clearance of upland forests to supply timber and cash-crops. At the same time, many Europeans had begun to attribute *paludismo* to parasites found in the human blood that could be passed on through mosquitoes. The term malaria came into more popular use across Europe and America and action was taken to target the parasites directly, largely through waging destruction on the habitats of the forest-dwelling mosquitoes that harboured them.

As the insect-ridden forest was implicated as the source of deadly fever, felling trees was consequently perceived by many in the colonial administration to also be an effective way of ridding the environment from pestilence (De Bevoise, 1995). Precisely the reverse happened as, crucially, this economic activity set huge swathes of people into motion, moving between sparsely populated upland forested areas where malaria parasites had circulated at 'stable' levels and lowland areas where the majority of inhabitants had, up until then, lived out of reach of the weak mosquito vectors and the parasites they carried. The subsequent deadly

---

[2] Written colonial accounts suggest the Spanish referred to Indigenous People as '*Indio*', the offspring of Spanish & *Indio* parents as '*Mestizos*', Spanish born in the Philippines as '*Filipino or Insulares*', and Spanish born in the Peninsula as '*Peninsulares*'.

exchange of disease-carrying pathogens among these now mobile, more densely packed and non-immune collections of people was exacerbated by the loss of almost the entire population of cattle and carabao (domestic water buffalo) to the rinderpest virus. Instead of biting their favoured bovine creatures, the *A. minimus flavirostris* mosquitoes turned on the newly abundant human hosts around them. Thus, the price of Spanish economic activity was that the ecological equilibrium between human, mosquito and parasite was tipped in favour of the latter. Fever surged and became the biggest killer in the late nineteenth-century Philippines amongst Indigenous populations and colonisers alike. While the threat to life and livelihood may well have played a part in spurring popular support for revolution against the Spanish, the disease was yet again implicated in a new colonial power's attempts to conquer and then oppress Indigenous People once more.

This shift in the power of parasites from relative protector to mass killer and oppressor of upland Indigenous People was heightened under Unites States (US) occupation, and coincided with the proliferation of ideas of germ theory. During this period (1898–1946), the colonial mission was guided by President William McKinley's strategy of 'benevolent assimilation'. The increasing use of biomedicine (the legacy of which is still present today) had the effect (or purpose, as some argue) of rationalising the 'white man's burden' overseas by transforming the islands into healthy, habitable places for US citizens to conduct their so-called civilisation of the 'savages' in safety (Anderson, 1992). As such, the scale-up of medical science and biomedicine and the systematic approach taken to targeting malaria parasites became an important component of colonial legitimacy and power. Malaria was implicated yet again in strategies of control and oppression. What becomes clear is that to understand the power of parasites, it is necessary to understand the human practices that surrounded them. By situating malaria in the context of these encounters, I demonstrate how parasites lost and gained power in the islands due to the very human relations and practices enacted in their name.

Malaria as Protector: Parasites in the Pre-colonial Era

From an epidemiological point of view, human malaria arises from a complex series of ecological interactions between parasites, mosquitoes and humans. Before the Spanish descended on the Philippines, parasites were likely circulating within the human population but are thought to have been largely confined to upland forested areas where only a small minority of the population lived. De Bevoise (1995) describes epidemics as an excessive, sudden enlargement or growth of 'what exists normally *in* … people so as to become something visited *upon* them' (ibid., p. 7). Consequently, it is necessary to situate the late nineteenth-century lethal dance between parasites, their vectors and hosts, in historical ecological context.

Anthropologists have long pointed out how an historical method is crucial for avoiding the synchronicity of some ethnographic studies that represent cultures without reference to time (Boas, 1896). An interactive perspective (i.e., one that has been both diachronic and synchronic aspects) is particularly important when referring to a group of people whose more recent history is intimately bound with colonialism and whose pre-colonial culture has been systematically denied in much historical Euro-American thought and academia (Cannell, 1999). For example, the Philippines has been described with authority as a country devoid of a 'social backbone' and as being merely imitative of two sets of Western colonisers, first Catholic Spain (1565–1898) and then Secular America (1898–1946) (ibid.). This distortion and obliteration of history in some Euro-American academic literature has meant that Filipinos have mistakenly and pejoratively been described as having no 'evocative era prior to the Spanish period to which [they] can now turn to with pride' (Steinberg, 1990, p. 54). In reality, archaeological, Indigenous and oral evidence unsurprisingly demonstrate the existence of a rich and established pre-colonial culture that, far from being isolated or insular, involved extensive foreign links (Junker, 1999). Alongside this long history of social complexity, movement and exchange, in terms of infectious diseases, evidence suggests that those such as malaria, dengue and schistosomiasis had all likely become established in the islands and spread along trade routes with China, Borneo, the Celebes and the Moluccas (McNeill, 1979; Newson, 1999) long before European colonisers arrived.

Despite being present in the pre-colonial context, the limited impact on humans was owed in large part to pre-colonial social organisation. Records suggest that when the Spanish invaded, population levels were relatively low at around 1.2 million, and only up to a thousand islands were inhabited (ibid.). Settlements were generally in lowland areas, with discontinuous clusters of houses hugging the rivers and the sea coast. It is important to note that pre-Hispanic settlements have often been homogenised in historical and academic accounts and collectively referred to as *barangays*—described as small clusters of related kin groups (20–100 people) living under the jurisdiction of a Chief or *datu* with the rest of the community consisting of *maharlika/timaua* (warriors or freed people) and debt-bond slaves (Rafael, 2018). According to Junker (1999), *datus* were able to maintain their status by providing for their village in three interrelated ways: trading (organising labour around the extraction and exchange of local goods); raiding (capturing goods and slaves from other communities); and feasting (redistributing wealth). However, this catch-all characterisation is unlikely to reflect the true variation among the vast numbers of ethno-linguistic groups across the islands. For one thing, the term *datu* has Malay roots—a position and related social order that no doubt was brought to the islands with the flow of Arab and Malay traders to the southern islands dating back as early as the twelfth century. Through his analysis of surviving texts written in Indigenous languages, historian Damon Woods (2017)[3] aims to give 'voice' to what he describes as the 'silenced' populations of the islands and attributes the homogenisation of social organisation in written records to colonial error. In particular, he notes the influence of one account, *Las costumbres de los indios Tagalog de Filipinas*, by the Franciscan friar Juan e Plasencia, on the characterisation by the colonial administration and their subsequent reorganisation of society. The lingering repercussions of these changes on Pälawan communities are discussed further in Chap. 4. For now, the point is that,

---

[3] The term *balangay* or *barangay* refers to a lashed-lug boat used as trading ships in the islands up until the colonial era.

regardless of the likely variation in social organisation, evidence suggests the majority of the population across the islands appeared to live in the lowlands with only around 10% residing in the upland forests alongside malaria parasites (Keesing, 1962).

Building archaeological and ethnohistorical evidence suggests that politically complex and socially stratified communities were found across the archipelago *before* luxury foreign goods were circulated through China and India in the early first millennium A.D. (Junker, 1999). Pre-colonial populations were therefore by no means living in 'aseptic isolation' (De Bevoise, 1995), instead mutually relying on fish, salt metals and ceramics from the shore and rice, cotton and forest products from the mountains, as well as engaging in overland exchange of products such as rice, sailcrafts, porcelain and people between islands. However, groups were nevertheless relatively limited in size and spread with the majority of contact between them made by water rather than overland. The transmission of widespread disease across the archipelago was consequently held back by a combination of seawater, distance, monsoon winds and the threat of pirates (De Bevoise, 1995; Newson, 1999). Outbreaks of human malaria were likely rare, seasonal, localised and self-limiting and the population on the whole was not at 'serious demographic risk from widespread epidemic disease' (De Bevoise, 1995, p. 17). In upland areas, although outbreaks would have caused high mortality among the small numbers of Indigenous populations residing there, these were rare and most afflicted people would have sadly died before they could pass on infection to others in high numbers (Newson, 1999). For those few who avoided death, relapses or recrudescence were no doubt common for periods of up to about five years, depending on the species of *Plasmodium*. This would have resulted in anaemia from the sustained destruction of infected red cells. However, over time, a certain level of acquired immunity would have been gained, protecting the surviving population from the most devastating and long-term effects of parasitic disease.

By contrast, although the exact levels of acquired immunity are unknown (McNeill, 1979), it is likely to have been inconsequential in the bulk of the lowland population where malaria was uncommon and unstable (De Bevoise, 1995). Lowlanders would have only rarely ventured into upland areas and thus had little opportunity to build up exposure and resistance. If some individuals did develop immunity from small-scale or one-off infections that they survived, they would have been anomalies rather than the norm. In most places around the world where malaria is endemic (constantly present), it tends to be concentrated in lowland areas (De Bevoise, 1995). The fact that it was the reverse in the Philippines meant that the majority of people were able to live below the endemic line, near the shore and away from mosquito vectors in most places where they lived. In this sense, *plasmodia*, and its concentration in the upland areas, presented Indigenous pre-colonial populations living there a lethal but relatively exceptional level of threat. It even arguably offered some protection for these groups against the colonial interference and invasion that was about to be unleashed on the archipelago.

Malaria as Killer: Parasites During Spanish Rule

By the end of 350 years of Spanish occupation, infectious diseases across the islands were rife. Cholera, beriberi, dysentery, tuberculosis, smallpox, typhoid fever, measles, rheumatic fevers, influenza, whooping cough, meningitis, diphtheria and tetanus had all increased to unprecedented levels. However, it was *paludismo* that was reported as the leading cause of mortality and morbidity year in and year out by Spanish physicians up until the end of their occupation (De Bevoise, 1995). History, and indeed all academic writing, can present a seamless narrative of events and circumstances, that no matter how complex, come together in a way that 'makes sense' of things and explains how they came about. This is especially true when reconstructed through written colonial records. Through the eyes (and reports) of the colonisers, fever was simply an innate part of the environment and the *Indios* that lived there, both of which they sought to 'civilise'. However, what becomes clear is that colonial practices were in fact the primary driving force behind *paludismo* having caused such devastation, that in the end also presented huge obstacles to the Spanish themselves. Although a growing body of critical post-colonial literature illustrates how the 'struggle and negotiation' of colonialism results from many 'murky and complex practical interactions' (Pels, 1997, p. 163) that are often excluded or obscured in official records, the fact remains that there is little in the way of documentary evidence relating to disease from the point of view of the colonised at all. Consideration of this period through the lens of what remains in Spanish documents (dating back to 1565) is therefore the predominant arena from which to base interpretation. While it will inevitably be incomplete and partial, it nevertheless illuminates some of the motivations, negotiations, dynamics and struggles that led to such disastrous ecological changes by the end of Spain's rule.

While prior European voyages may have taken place, records document that in 1521, Portuguese explorer Ferdinand Magellan landed on a group of islands in the western *Pacific* Ocean during his expedition on behalf of King Charles 1 of Spain. This was part of the sixteenth-century competition (mainly with Portugal) to extract resources such as gold and spices that were thought to be abundant in *Las Islas del Poniente*[4] (Constantino & Constantino, 2008) and, crucially, in the race to Christianise unexplored regions to the East as part of Charles' vision of establishing a religious 'Oriental Empire' (Tan, 1987). Shortly after seeking alliances with leaders of the central islands, Magellan was killed on the island of Mactan by the troops of Lapu-Lapu who successfully resisted and overturned conquest. Subsequent expeditions continued however, and in 1543, explorer Ruy Lopez de Villalobos named the islands *las islas Filipinas* (Rafael, 2018) after heir apparent, Felipe II. In 1565, accompanied by five Augustinian friars, navigator Miguel López de Legazpi found a return route between New Spain (Mexico) and the Spice Islands, making the Philippines a useful conduit in between. He therefore set up a permanent Spanish outpost in Manila in 1571 by forcibly evicting its rulers and inhabitants before rebuilding the new capital in the Spanish 'style' with a cathedral, plaza and public offices. Only *Peninsulares* (peninsular Spanish) were allowed to reside within this walled city while *Indios were largely re*settled outside. This set in motion the takeover of most of the coastal and lowland areas of the archipelago from Luzon to northern Mindanao which had fallen under Spanish control by the end of the century. Although some of Magellan's original fleet did land on the island of Palawan following his death, or 'The Land of Promise' as they called it,

---

[4] Spanish term for the East Indies from the Philippines to New Guinea.

they were met with fierce resistance from ruling Tausug communities[5] who managed to maintain their grip on the areas until as late as 1749 when the Sultanate of Sulu—a Muslim polity with its capital in Jolo island—eventually surrendered the island. By 1818, the entirety of Paragua (as it was then called) was organised as a single province renamed Calamianes, with its capital established in Taytay[6] in the north which was similarly subject to Spanish reorganisation as they had managed to take control of the seas by establishing a naval station in Puerto Princesa in 1872 (Macdonald, 2007). However, in reality, it seems the Sultanate never really relinquished control of the southern coastlines, integrating trading centres into the 'Sulu zone' which Warren (1981) describes as a Southeast Asian economic region composed of ethnically and politically heterogeneous societies until well into the twentieth century. Unable to completely take control of Southern Palawan, the Spanish left Tausug *datus* free to exploit Indigenous People by pushing some further into the fever-ridden forests and extracting yearlong supplies of tribute rice, forest products such as beeswax, honey, rattan and resin as well as labour from the uplands to send to Jolo island (ibid.). Crucially however, the forested hills and mountains of Southern Palawan remained relatively sparsely populated and untouched by *datus* who took no real interest in either transforming or governing them (Smith, 2020).

In the rest of the colony, unlike in their occupation of Latin America, Spanish interest in the Philippines was token in economic terms up until the late-nineteenth century (Cannell, 1999). Historian Tan (1987) summarises the aims of Spanish colonisation as God, Glory and Gold based on his analysis of written records. The Philippines had no spices of value, and being geographically remote from Spain[7] was regarded merely as a channel to better things, rather than being important in its own right. The islands were essentially considered a sub-colony of the empire in

---

[5] Rafael (2018) documents how Islam came to the islands in the mid-twelfth century, quite late for the region and the rest of the world, by way of Arab traders and Malay missionaries. Its spread was confined to the southern tip of the archipelago in places such as Palawan, Mindanao and the Sulu Archipelago leaving only faint marks further north, especially around Manila.

[6] The current capital Puerto Princesa was established as capital in 1872.

[7] Distance was compounded by an ancient agreement between Portugal and Spain that meant the Spanish route to the Philippines was via the Americas.

New Spain. The port of Manila was closed to all but New Spain and acted as a thoroughfare for the galleon trade passing Eastern, especially Chinese, silk to Acapulco in exchange for Latin American silver (Cannell, 1999). Distance from Spain discouraged many *Peninsulares* from settling in the colony and they made up less than 1% of the population (Rafael, 2018). Conversely, many more Mexican Creoles or Latin American Mestizos migrated there and took up low-level professional positions (Steinberg, 1990) with some Mexican convicts also exiled to the islands from recruiting centres and jails and forced into labour under the *forzado* system (Mawson, 2013; Mehl, 2016). Non-Han southern Chinese traders provided services such as carpentry, masonry and printing and acted as the middlemen in trade with New Mexico (Rafael, 2018). Due to the heavy subsidies being paid by the Mexican treasury to support the colony, the merchants of Seville wanted to abandon the 'poor' islands altogether but were met with opposition from religious officials who were keen to hold on to it as their 'warehouse of Christianity' in the East (Camba, 2012). In fact, with so few *Peninsulares* willing to relocate, Spain came to rely heavily on its friars as *de facto* administrators of the islands so much so that they turned, in time, from acting as 'guardians' of *Indios* against harsh treatment from soldiers to becoming their dominant oppressors.

The factors that led to an increase in fever rates during the long rule of the Spanish are complex and multi-faceted. As described above, pre-colonial settlement patterns meant that, socially as well as physically, the population at large was impermeable to significant infection. As De Bevoise (1995) puts it, this 'island world comprised archipelagos within an archipelago, islands within islands' (ibid., p. 18) and offered some level of protection against the spread of large-scale epidemics. However, significant changes to land-use, the means of production and social organisation ensued, as the people I met in Palawan were all too aware of. As an older member of the Pälawan community, Reso, told me:

> Before outsiders came to this island, our *kagurangurangan* (ancestors) lived sometimes by the shoreline or up in the mountains and used the land up there [indicating the upland areas] for growing rice since time immemorial. The land was passed down to us from them. They would clear a small patch

and then pass some of it to their children when they got married, saying 'this place from the banana tree over there until this *kalamansi* lime tree here is now yours and you can take anything that grows here'. So we did not need to have anything to do with the authorities. Land was just like that. But when the Muslims and then the Christians came, things changed. The Christians especially said 'This land and these trees or this banana grove is not yours and you can't just take from it like before'. From that time on, our ancestors had to move to live very high in the mountains or down here where the land belonged to someone else. It is not how it was in the past when we were scattered all around. From that time on, people were hungrier and sicker because they could not do their own farming and they started to get diseases brought from outsiders.

Although these changes were enforced much later across Southern Palawan due to the resistance to the Spanish by the Tausugs, as Reso describes, land was re-classified across the archipelago and communal allocation gave way to private ownership. The Regalian Doctrine was imposed, stipulating that any non-privately owned land and natural resources were now deemed 'public domain' (i.e., possession of the Crown) (Lynch, 2011). An *encomienda* (labour) system was imposed by Governor Miguel López de Legazpi, beginning in Manila, encouraging soldiers and clergy to apply for titles and the right to collect an annual tribute from tenants. *Reducción* was introduced as a policy to forcibly relocate all *Indios* into the lowlands to provide *polos y servicios* (forced labour) giving men (except those from elite groups who were required to collect taxes and labour instead) of working age (16–60) no choice but to surrender their labour for at least 40 days a year to work the land for its new 'owners' (Cannell, 1999; Rafael, 2018).[8] Friars marched together with soldiers, the cross an essential companion to the sword, and the Spanish clergy assumed increasingly control with the Dominicans, Franciscans, Recollects and Jesuits that followed the Augustinians acting as both religious and secular authority (ibid.).

---

[8] *Polos y servicios* was major reason why African slavery was absent from the Philippines as it provided surplus labour plus it would have been a considerable cost to ship slaves to the islands due to their location (Rafael, 2018).

Communities were thus reorganised and unrelated groups of people brought together in denser constellations in an attempt to impose administrative convenience and to bring people 'under the bells' of the church (ibid.). In return, for their pacification and submission to the Crown, converts were provided religious instruction and some material benefit (Santiago, 1990). However, the population was essentially bifurcated into those who were deemed 'productive' (Christians) and therefore eligible for land titles due to their status as closer to God and those who were considered 'primitive' (*Indios*) and ineligible for such Grace. As is discussed in more detail in Chap. 4, changes to land and the upland/lowland Christian/native distinctions that began here and eventually spread to Southern Palawan endured at the time of my fieldwork and continued to have consequences for Indigenous Peoples who were still facing considerable obstacles to gaining land titles for their ancestral domains. As Santiago (1990) describes, venerable records at the Archivo General de Indias in Sevilla, Spain, suggested as little as ten Filipino *Indios* had become *encomenderos* (grant holders) in the seventeenth and early eighteenth centuries and for the majority of the population, *encomenderos* were known to overwork their tenants and place heavy demands on them (Cannell, 1999, p. 5). There were indeed accounts of revolts, with some churches being burnt down and inhabitants refusing to settle, with those who refused to comply with the tribute system killed, imprisoned or had their villages pillaged and burnt. Those who escaped such fates fled, were forced into hiding or banished into what were perceived as the inhabitable, fever-ridden uplands. Lowland settlements were concentrated around lowland *pueblos* (towns) containing the *poblacion* (administrative centre), the church, a market, town hall and major houses (De Bevoise, 1995). What is significant is that this combination of increased concentration and movement between densely and sparsely populated areas in this reorganisation period led to the inevitable spread of pestilence and disease including *paludismo*.

In terms of available remedies, Joven (2012) explains how limited medical supplies were available through the annual Manila-Acapulco Galleon Trade in which provisions were requested from Manila as well as some from China. European-trained physicians, surgeons and pharmacists were limited to Manila and serviced only the government and its

workers. Religious orders supported pioneering natural history and astro-
nomical research from the sixteenth and seventeenth centuries onwards,
establishing hospitals in Manila and Cavite that acted as refuges for the
poor. However, in more provincial areas, it was local *curanderos* or
mediquillos[9] who mainly serviced the population through a combination
of plant-based treatments, massage and hydrotherapy. Despite being dismissed as 'quacks' and frowned upon for their 'superstitious' beliefs, missionaries and parish priests simultaneously sought alliances with
curanderos in order to learn their remedies that they did acquiesce were
highly effective. Over time, Joven (2012) documents how a unique and
state-of-the-art medical and pharmaceutical science developed out of this
collaboration and resulted in the publication of many books on Philippine
pharmacopoeia that priests intended for use among local populations.[10]
While the clergy never came round to fully condoning what they saw as
the 'devilish' belief systems that underpinned their teachers' practices,
they were able to secularise it enough to make it palatable to ecclesiastical
authorities and therefore fill the gap created by the lack of other medical
professionals and supplies from the administration. As Anderson (2007)
explains, from the eighteenth century onwards a more complex entanglement between religion and secular medical practices emerged as the
Spanish Enlightenment increasingly cast scepticism on religious doctrine,
advocating instead the detached observation encouraged by the likes of
Montesquieu, Voltaire, Rousseau and Diderot. While this had some
effect in the Philippines, the clergy by and large continued to incorporate
and use scientific endeavours that, although subordinate to confession,
were also considered a route to personal salvation. Many governors therefore continued to promote research in agriculture and botany as a way of
alleviating suffering from the diseases afflicting colonisers and colonised
alike in high numbers.

The intentional changes to land ownership that caused such hardship
and sickness for many *Indios* were accompanied by other destabilising

---

[9] According to Joven (2012), the Spaniards used the umbrella term '*curandero*' to refer to the local
traditional healers and 'were sometimes interchangeably referred to as *mediquillos*, a generic term
applied to individuals who had a trickling of western medical training and experience, could pre-
scribe medicines, but devoid of the supernatural healing features' (ibid., p. 175).

[10] See Joven (2012) for a comprehensive list.

forces. The Spanish-Dutch wars broke out in 1609 as Holland rebelled over commercial supremacy in the spice-rich Moluccas. In order to finance the wars, the colonial administration used *polo y servicios* to set thousands of subjects to fell timber, build—and sail—ships and man guns. In addition, through *vandala* (forced sale of produce), they requisitioned supplies to clothe and feed their men. Furthermore, by their peak in the third quarter of the eighteenth century, raids on southern islands in Luzon and the Visayas by the Tausug from Mindanao and the Sulu Archipelago were threatening life and wellbeing even further. Reversing the trend of Christian raids on their own lands, the Tausug burnt houses and crops, cut down fruit trees and slaughtered animals across the archipelago (De Bevoise, 1995, p. 21). The negative effects of both population settlement/increase and raids on public health should not be minimised (ibid.). Together, these radical social and economic shifts under Spanish rule meant settlements and everyday life was unstable and extremely difficult.

The hardship of the Dutch wars ended in 1648 and a population upsurge occurred that would continue to 'shape the health crises two centuries later' (ibid., p. 23). During this time of peace, colonial rule did play a part in bringing about an end to inter-*barangay* warfare and a minimisation of the raids from the Muslim south. The closed port in Manila did also have the effect of limiting the importation of external parasites. Under such conditions, birth rates rose steeply and the population increased, reaching a peak in 1840 (De Bevoise, 1995). However, while 'the effect of colonial rule in this period was to nurture life, [it was also] simultaneously to destroy it [as] periods of imperial peace were built on [the] suffering and death of so many' (ibid.). As De Bevoise (1995) states, what ensued next was not random, but the result of a range of administrative, geographic, cultural and economic factors. In other words, it was of human making.

The demographic changes of the late nineteenth century that wreaked such epidemiological havoc largely came about due to substantial economic reform instigated because of the colony's changing role in the faltering Spanish Empire. As described above, an economy based on subsistence agriculture and the production of handcrafted goods was of little interest to the Spanish when they first arrived (De Bevoise, 1995).

However, the collapse of Spanish rule in Latin America ended the galleon trade in the early nineteenth century (Steinberg, 1990), and as Spain lost ground, the Philippines seemed increasingly like an 'unaffordable luxury' (De Bevoise, 1995, p. 27). No longer sustained by silver from Mexican mines, Spain began to abandon the view of the Philippines as a 'conduit to other things' (Steinberg, 1990, p. 54) and embarked on a radical programme of economic investment to transform the fertile islands into a support system for the Empire. By royal decree, the Philippines was turned into a producer and exporter of timber and cash-crops in order to prevent the demise of foreign interest in trade and prevent the loss of the colony (De Bevoise, 1995). The port of Manila was opened in 1834 to external trade mainly from Europe and the United States.

Initially, lush, upland forests were opened up in an attempt to make the Philippines the principal Far Eastern market for timber (De Bevoise, 1995, p. 142). In 1855, the Inspección de Montes was established and charged with the exploration and survey of mountains, forests and lands. In less than a decade, it took over active management of Indigenous forest lands. However, De Bevoise (1995), documents how, by the end of the century, the expected revenue from timber was not as demonstrable as the wealth generated from cash-cropping and so opposition mounted against the Inspección. Those that advocated cultivation advanced a new line of argument—that the mass felling of trees was also necessary to promote good health. For example, the secretary of the agriculture board, Manuel del Busto, lauded the successes of colonists the world over who had succeeded in clearing fever-ridden forests using Puerto Princesa in Palawan, as a local case in point. Whereas only six inhabitants had been free of fevers in 1877, now almost all were rid of any such suffering, he proclaimed (ibid.). In time, those who favoured cash-cropping over managed conservation triumphed and resources were allocated accordingly. Reserved forest lands were to be kept to a minimum and cultivated lands were instead developed in cleared areas. Land therefore became an increasingly profitable commodity especially upland, fertile areas. Vast numbers of people were now thrown into motion, moving between endemic upland areas and 'healthier' lowland areas in new ways. Early pioneers paid a heavy price for this. As non-immune populations entered uphill endemic zones to fell trees and cultivate land, their non-immune blood provided substantial new reservoirs of infection (De Bevoise, 1995). The price for this economic activity was that the equilibrium between parasite, mosquito and human was disturbed and malaria consequently surged at the expense of thousands of human lives.

The situation was equally dire in provincial islands such as Palawan. The arrival of the steam ship in the mid-1800s meant that during this period of cash-cropping proliferation, a whole host of migrants working with large trading companies of China, the United States and Europe flocked to the Philippines as merchant bankers, paying advances for crops such as sugar, copra, tobacco, coffee and hemp (Steinberg, 1990). Once Spain had been expelled from Latin America, many more *Peninsulares* also fled to Manila, taking over professional positions from the *Mestizos* (children born from (usually) Filipina mothers and either Spanish or Chinese fathers) who had been successful in agricultural production and export. Being pushed out of trade activities from many directions, these *Mestizos* often moved to frontier provinces such as Palawan, particularly in the north, to try their luck at commercial agriculture, becoming, for the first time, 'real hacendados' (Anderson, 1988, p. 7) of the island. The deficient land title system meant they were able to take advantage, moving into areas on unprecedented scales to acquire titles to land that was now so profitable and pushing yet more Indigenous People into the uplands. These new inhabitants cleared trees, often next to streams, to make way for their homes and farms in areas that were prime locations for *A. minimus flavirostris* to thrive. With an abundance of non-immune hosts to bite and ample indoor nocturnal resting places, the mosquitoes and parasites that they carried flourished.

As mentioned above, another crucial facilitator fuelling *paludismo* epidemics in the nineteenth century was the loss of around 90% of cattle and carabao to rinderpest disease from 1888 onwards. De Bevoise (1995) describes the importation of the virus (suspected to be from Indochina) to the islands as 'arguably the single greatest catastrophe in nineteenth-century Philippines' (ibid., p. 158). The loss meant there was no way of tilling and farmers were unable to cultivate land, reducing food supplies and exacerbating malnutrition and debt. To make matters worse, untilled land was a desirable breeding ground for mosquitoes, and without their favoured cattle to feed on, the abundant mosquitoes feasted on humans instead, sparking seasonal lethal epidemics on top of hunger and poverty throughout 1888–1889. Not only did disease surge but agricultural output was set back for years, with hundreds of people too sick to work and no cattle to turn the fields.

It is no surprise, then, that against this backdrop the colonial administration had increasingly realised the importance of public health in the governance of the colony, but they began to put a particular emphasis on preventive care for only certain diseases through vaccination (Anderson, 2006). Spain had ordered mandatory immunisation in her colonies from 1806 and the central board of vaccination in Manila was producing and distributing smallpox inoculations for example. This interventionalist approach did however have a knock-on effect for *paludismo* as it prompted the establishment of the first secular medical school in Manila in 1871 in the Catholic University of Santo Tomas (UST) (despite some opposition by the religious establishment), with faculties of medicine, surgery and pharmacy. Courses in infectious diseases led to students being sent out across the islands to collect and return statistics on disease cases including *paludismo*. However, the focus of such institutions was firmly in ensuring the public health of the colony and academic studies were not possible. Instead, doctoral candidates had to enrol in European universities for this. Many who did so were the native-borne children of the elite merchant classes of *Insulares*, *Mestizos* and *Indios* who had prospered enough to afford the expense of the Universidad Central de Madrid (Vallejo, 2017). Included in this group of *Ilustrados* (the enlightened) was Antonio Luna whose family had made their fortune in tobacco. Whilst in Spain, he became an active member of the Propaganda, a reform movement of Filipino expatriates in Madrid which was organised into a cohesive group by 1886. Although Luna is often remembered for his military career and fierce character, given the prominent role he later played in the revolution, less attention has been paid to his scientific career and, in particular, how his work on malaria intertwined with his political sentiments. As Vallejo (2017) described, Luna, along with other prominent scholars, was sent by the colonial government to complete his doctorate at the Universidad Central de Madrid in 1983, on the condition he return to the Philippines to head the public health bureaucracy that was increasingly seen as instrumental in tackling infectious disease and legitimising colonial power. This period coincided with a shift in European scientific thinking away from ideas of environmental causes of tropical infections towards emerging notions of germ theory influenced by those such as Louis Pasteur and Robert Koch. Luna's own thesis, '*El hematozoario del paludismo: su estudio experimental*', was published as a treatise in 1893 and focused on forms of *paludismo*[11] in human blood, relating these to the symptoms fever, chills and the enlargement of the spleen and liver. His interest lay in determining when the best time would be to administer quinine—the active ingredient found in the South American evergreen shrub, cinchona, that Quechua people had been using to treat fevers and chills for hundreds of years. Luna's work was fundamental in informing the gold standard for malaria diagnostics that is still used today, the blood film method. Crucially, at the time, his parasite studies particularly influenced the work of Italian malariologists Giovanni Battista Grassi, Amico Bignami, Giuseppe Bastianelli, Angelo Celli, Camillo Golgi and Ettore Marchiafava who, in 1989, concluded that there was enough evidence to suggest parasites were transmitted to humans by mosquitoes, specifically *anophelines* that, a British officer, Ronald Ross had observed carried parasites in their gut, undermining hypotheses relating to environmental causes of malaria from 'bad air'.

On his return to the Philippines, Luna was appointed Municipal Chemist of the City of Manila. He was therefore part of the moves by colonial powers to establish a health infrastructure that was, to some extent, successful. By the end of Spanish rule, all provinces of the country except one had a *medico titular* or a government physician with quarantine systems in place and municipal chemistry and bacteriology laboratories established (Vallejo, 2017). Significantly, the scientific 'objectivity' that Luna argued for in his quest to enable Filipinos to diagnose malaria was also applied to his views on Filipino autonomy within the Spanish metropolis. For Propagandists like him, independence would be achieved by careful, rational, negotiated reform proposals with Spain. It is well documented that the prominent Propagandist and 'National Hero' José

---

[11] Luna preferred not to use the term 'malaria' following the French military physician Charles Laveran in using '*paludismo*'. Stationed in Constantine, Algeria in 1880, Laveran observed parasites in the blood of soldiers suffering from fever and was of the opinion that 'malaria' has a superstitious etymology and was unsuitable in scientific work (Bruce-Chwatt, 1981).

Rizal studied medicine in Europe and is said to have developed a similar commitment to objectivity and reason that informed his politics. For him, patriotism implied a scientific orientation to the world. While scientists such as Luna and Rizal were fundamental in spurring the revolution, the Filipino historian Reynaldo Ileto (1979) has argued that lower-class Filipinos were equally influential and may have used recourse to religion rather than the science of the elites as their impetus for bottom-up revolution. Specifically, the *awit* (Tagalog verse) and *pabasa* (sung performance) that relate to the suffering and death of Christ—or what is known as the *Pasyon* (Passion)—was potentially used as way of making sense of and ultimately articulating rebellion to colonial rule. Bucking the scholarly trend of attributing change only to the educated *Ilustrados* he suggests instead that the *Pasyon* provided the lower classes with idioms through which to articulate and form a religiously guided class consciousness that manifested in a series of uprisings from 1840 to 1910 and that greatly influenced the nationalistic movement. In more immediate terms, as malaria shifted from protecting small clusters of Indigenous populations from colonial control to killing them in huge numbers that had never been seen before across the islands, Filipinos were faced with severe threats to their physical, economic, social and political lives. In his critique of Ileto (1979), Scalice (2018) suggests instead that revolutionaries successfully appealed to the urban working class of predominately agricultural labourers by offering a practical and concrete way out of the severe economic and social hardship they faced, with rebellion lying far beyond the sphere of religious salvation. It is perhaps no wonder then that while fever raged in the settlements, revolution filled the air. In 1896, Spanish authorities discovered the secret anti-colonial Katipunan (revolutionary society) who subsequently declared a nationwide revolution with their leader Andrés Bonifacio calling for an attack on Manila. Following a series of provincial revolts across the colony, a power struggle ensued among the revolutionaries culminating in Bonifacio's execution in 1897 and command shifting to Emilio Aguinaldo. However, Aguinaldo signed the Pact of Biak-na-Bato with Spain's colonial Governor-General Fernando Primo de Rivera on 15 December 1987, bringing hostilities and revolution to a temporary end. Aguinaldo and a group of loyal Filipino officers, upheld as both heroes and villains, the 'brains of the nation' who began but then 'betrayed' the revolution, exiled themselves in the British colony of Hong Kong and established the Hong Kong Junta. Two years later however, Aguinaldo was contacted by the Americans who promised him independence for his Republic in return for his help bringing down Spanish rule.

Malaria as Oppressor: Parasites During the American Occupation

On Sunday 24 April 1898, Hon. Spencer Pratt, the US Consul-General to Singapore, received a telegraph from Admiral Dewey, the US *Commodore*, who was stationed in Hong Kong, awaiting orders to invade the Philippines. 'Tell Aguinaldo come soon as possible', he wrote to Pratt, who had successfully tracked down the Filipino revolutionary in Singapore (Worcester, 1921). Aguinaldo had arrived only days before, *incognito* and accompanied by a small group of insurgents. By the time Pratt received conformation to try to persuade the exiled revolutionary to help bring down the Spanish, triggered by activity in Cuba and their war of independence from Spain, American President McKinley had already signed the Joint Resolution to go to war with the European power. The ten-week Spanish-American war of 1898 culminated in the defeat of the Spanish at the Battle of Manila Bay, and in the peace Treaty of Paris, signed in December that year, the US agreed to pay Spain $20,000,000 for the islands in recognition of the loss of their public buildings and public works. Although Aguinaldo had declared the Philippines a provisional republic six months before in June 1898, the hopes of the new President and his revolutionaries were clearly quashed as McKinley had no intention of facilitating Independence, and the First Philippine Republic went unrecognised by both Spain and the United States. Rid of one set of brutal colonisers, the islands were under takeover by another. In 1899, the Republic declared war on the United States with Filipinos resorting to guerrilla warfare. The Americans saw this as insurgency and proof of the racial inferiority of what they referred to as the 'injuns' and 'niggers'

(Rafael, 2018). The fight degenerated into a cruel war of extermination with the United States as Rafael (2018) describes:

> American troops burned villages to deprive guerrillas of support, herding inhabitants into concentration camps. They executed prisoners and any males suspected of being an insurgent as young as ten years old. They routinely engaged in torture, especially in the water cure, and as with all armies of occupation, raped, pillaged, and plundered their way across the archipelago. (ibid.)

As Aguinaldo's commander-in-chief, Antonio Luna played a prominent role in the fight, but in the end, it led not only to his murder in 1899, due to a breakdown in his relations with Aguinaldo, but also to the total collapse of the public health system that he had established under Spanish rule. Two years later, Aguinaldo himself was captured by the Americans and eventually pledged allegiance to them. For the second time, the 'heroes' of the nation surrendered their homeland. For the rest of his life Aguinaldo wore a black bow tie in public to mourn the loss of the Republic, only stopping in 1946, following independence. By 1902 the war had ended and the Americans took over the islands at the expense of between 250,000 and 1 million Filipino lives and 4000 American ones. Most of the deaths had occurred from wounds, famine and, of course, infectious fever.

President McKinley declared his strategy in the Philippines to be one guided by 'benevolent assimilation' in what he described as an attempt to liberate, not subjugate, Filipinos through Christianisation, education and healthcare, eventually leading them to the path of self-governance. In the main, this was in order to depoliticise and demilitarise the independence movement through encouraging Filipino collaboration and participation in the colonial administration (Rafael, 2018) but was also a practical response to the devastating effects of years of fighting which had by now wreaked so much havoc across the islands. Once war between America and Spain had been declared in 1898, both sides had shipped thousands of foreign soldiers to the archipelago, bringing with them diseases from North America, Cuba, Hawaii and China. Once in the Philippines, soldiers also contracted Indigenous ailments, the most serious being fever.

Most American army medical officers were unaware of the links that were increasingly being made between fever, parasites and mosquitoes, still attributing the sickness that swarmed their ranks to 'exposure to the sun on the march' and the 'filth', 'mists' and 'vapours' that arose from the ground after a 'hard rain' (De Bevoise, 1995). De Bevoise (1995) recounts how war also fuelled another major outbreak of rinderpest among carabao. Transmission had been kept at bay following their decimation a decade earlier, but while they were unlikely to have been responsible for bringing the bovine virus to the islands again, the Americans certainly exacerbated this latest spread by requesting all the carabaos it could locate be used in haulage. Animals were now travelling together in large groups over much greater distances, easily spreading the disease by nasal discharge (ibid.). While the Americans were largely unmoved by the complete dissemination of animal life, switching instead to the large numbers of mules and horses that the imported into the islands, for Filipinos it meant that yet again they lost the animals that were so integral to their livelihoods and health. As De Bevoise (1995) explains:

> Malaria followed of course. No one seems to have had any new insight into the connection, however. If they had, presumably the U.S. Army command would not have encouraged its malaria-ridden troops to kill the remaining beasts as part of the pacification program. Nor would it have been indifferent to those who killed livestock just for fun. The ecological process was inexorable once mosquitos were deprived of their primary blood meals. (ibid., p. 162)

Combined with the collapse of Luna's health system, a public health crisis ensued among both soldiers and civilians that needed urgent attention if the new colonial powers were going to be able to assume any kind of authority. The very same fever that threatened Spanish dominance decades before was now implicated in America's subsequent ability to gain control over the islands.

To make matters worse, just as the Filipino-American war was coming to an end, as well as having to deal with famine, dysentery and fever of their own making to a large degree, a serious outbreak of cholera swept across the islands that too directly related to the social and environmental aftermath of war. Ileto (1995) argues that the subsequent US 'war' against cholera was barely differentiated from their 'pacification' of Filipinos, as a sanitary order that was ushered in response was a continuation of the act of war. Not only was the public health campaign of quarantine and sanitation discussed in similar military metaphorical terms but it was also operationalised through the militaristic burning of infected dwellings and the dispersal of gathered crowds. While ostensibly this was due to the risk of infection in line with contemporary ideas of germ theory, it was also used as a mechanism for dispelling potential sites of social and political critique.

The approach taken to cholera mirrored the American way of dealing with other infectious disease and similar attention was given to 'battling' malaria, smallpox, leprosy and the bubonic plague. While these afflicted Filipinos and US colonisers and thus deserved attention, those issues that affected Filipinos alone such as tuberculosis, infant mortality and the locally defined *beri-beri* (caused by vitamin B1 deficiency) were approached only after other diseases had been managed (McElhinny, 2005). In some cases, this effect (or purpose) of reducing the 'white man's burden' overseas by transforming the colony into a healthy, habitable city for American citizens was made explicit. For example, Sullivan (1991) refers to how American physician Victor Heiser alienated Filipinos by repeatedly citing improvement in public health as essential for increased US commercial activity in the Philippines. 'Diseased Orientals', he argued, posed a constant threat to Occidentals (cited in McElhinny, 2005). McElhinny (2005) describes how numerous tracts described Filipinos as children: 'highly impressionable, unable to reflect on their own conditions, and capable only of mimicking the actions of those above them' (ibid., p. 35).

A such, Rafael (2018) writes that the 'white Americans' conceived of colonisation as an open-ended tutelary relationship in which they acted as 'innately superior yet exceptionally benevolent masters of a wild collection of tribes of dark, brown, and mixed raced people yet to be tamed and pacified into a people who recognized their place in the new imperial order'. This appeared no more true than in the arena of colonial medicine as the microscope gave way to the sword (Anderson, 2007). Anderson (2007) documents how pretty much as soon as they arrived, the Americans set up biological laboratories and once they had established a civil government intensified this as a Bureau of Government Laboratories was set up at the behest of Dean Worcester, the secretary of the interior in the Philippine Commission, in order to consolidate all of the search activities of the colonial state (ibid.). By 1905 this was reorganised, expanded and renamed to the Bureau of Science and encompassed research and service units in tropical medicine, botany, zoology, entomology, chemistry and geology (ibid.). The Bureau's Philippine Journal of Science was launched in 1906 and soon became the leading science journal in the tropics. A medical school which reproduced the Johns Hopkins' emphasis on laboratory instruction and a hospital with modern laboratory facilities were also set up by the government. Biomedical science thrived under American occupation and 'before long, it seemed that the laboratory might reshape the lives of Filipinos as effectively as any religious ritual performed during the Spanish era' (Anderson, 2007, p. 303).

Anderson (1992) argues that American colonial science was established to investigate the 'truth' about the 'tropics' and by becoming the authoritative voice on these matters also acted as important components of colonial legitimacy. Over time, these laboratories helped render imperialism as simultaneously powerful and benign to some extent. By 1902, government laboratories namely the Bureau of Science and the Army Board for the Study of Tropical Diseases (housed within) conducted experiments to compare Filipino and American adaptations to the tropics. Initially, the environment was implicated as the main cause of diseases and ill-health and efforts were invested in helping colonisers to acclimatise to the 'wild' surroundings. Later, as biomedical ideas gained traction, attention shifted to the role of microbial pathogens within bodies. By the end of the first decade of the century, American physicians almost universally subscribed to germ theory and relationships between living beings were seen in the context of struggle for survival that could be overcome through knowledge and technology. In 1914, Andrew Balfour spoke to the London Society of Tropical Medicine and Hygiene and suggested that evidence had shown that 'by far the larger part of the morbidity and mortality in the Philippines [was] due to nostalgia, isolation, tedium, venereal disease, alcoholic excess, and especially to infections with various parasites' (Anderson, 1992, p. 506). This gave rise to a kind of aggressive warfare against disease-causing microbes (Ileto, 1995, p. 60).

Once parasites were implicated in the transmission of malaria, the Army Board in the Philippines set about diagnosing potentially malarious fevers and found that the parasites were commonly found in the blood of lowland Filipinos, especially children. Malaria and hookworm were established as the cause of anaemia and a host of other associated illnesses that were once attributed to the forest environment. Filipino bodies that contained parasites were thought to pose a threat to white bodies and needed to be controlled through strict sanitary regimes. Thus 'tropical science managed to convert the dirty, humid, teeming, complex environment into controllable specimens and measurements, which were further consolidated as figures in the scientific papers' (Anderson, 2004, p. 525). Safety for Americans would be achieved through restriction of contact with tropical fauna that now included Filipino bodies (ibid.). Similar to the cholera outbreak of 1902–1904, victory over disease became assimilated into the universal history of medical progress, torn from its original moorings in a colonial war and pacification campaign (Ileto, 1995). Control of water and food supplies, insect vectors and crucially colonial bodies who were now objects of medical science did contribute to keeping typhoid, cholera, yellow fever and crucially malaria in check (Anderson, 1992), but simultaneously and as a result, colonial laboratories played an important role in constituting Western physical and cultural authority as 'the economic and political aspects of American colonialism in the Philippines [were] rapidly … translated into the language of medical science' (Anderson, 1992, p. 507).

Conclusion

American control of the Islands ended in 1941 when the Japanese invaded and this Military Administration sought, unlike the Spanish and Americans before them, not to convert or assimilate the population but to economically and culturally subsume them into the so-called East Asia Co-Prosperity Sphere (Rafael, 2018). Invasion brought about the disintegration of Philippine scientific research and educational activities, hampering public health initiatives all over again. After the Japanese were forced out in 1945, and the Philippines finally gained independence in 1946, the Filipino elite, who now dominated in the field of science, had to rebuild local institutions from the ground up. Since the 1930s in particular, 'science was conventionally linked to nation building and the earlier American emphasis on its role in a more general civilizing mission now seemed redundant and insulting' (Anderson, 2007, p. 305). In this period of independence, science became increasingly justified in secular and economic terms and this sets the scene for the more contemporary context I discuss in the remainder of this book. In this chapter, I have focussed attention on the power of parasites particularly in the colonial period of the Philippines to stress how intimately linked this was to oppressive relations of power. However, as Rafael (2018) argues, while colonial rule rests on relations of power and persistent structures of inequality, it is also productive of new life forms, novel historical agents and ongoing social conflicts whose resolutions are still yet to come. As such, the enforced stability and coerced consensus of any imperial arrangement is always undermined and made more ambiguous. He writes that 'Janus-faced, the Philippines peers into the past of its imperial origins while looking out into the future of its post-colonial possibilities' (ibid.). It is to this post-colonial context that I turn to next to describe how malaria remained embroiled in the lives of more contemporary actors in Bataraza, presenting them with both obstacles and opportunities as they engaged in their own strategies to retain power within the different kinds in the 'fields' (Bourdieu, 1977) the colonisers left behind.

References

Anderson, B. (1988). Cacique democracy in the Philippines: Origins and dreams. *New Left Review*, *169*.

Anderson, W. (1992). "Where every prospect pleases and only man is vile": Laboratory medicine as colonial discourse. *Critical Inquiry*, *18*(3), 506–529. https://doi.org/10.1086/448643

Anderson, W. (2004). Natural histories of infectious disease: Ecological vision in twentieth-century biomedical science. *Osiris (Bruges)*, *19*, 39–61.

Anderson, W. (2006). *Colonial pathologies American tropical medicine, race, and hygiene in the Philippines / Warwick Anderson.* Duke University Press.

Anderson, W. (2007). Science in the Philippines. *Philippine Studies, 55*(3), 287–318. http://www.jstor.org/stable/42633917

Boas, F. (1896). The limitations of the comparative method of anthropology. *Science, 4*(103), 901–908. https://doi.org/10.1126/science.4.103.90

Bourdieu, P. (1977). *Outline of a theory of practice.* Cambridge University Press.

Bruce-Chwatt, L. J. (1981). Alphonse Laveran's discovery 100 years ago and today's global fight against malaria. *J R Soc Med. Jul, 74*(7), 531–536.

Camba, A. (2012). Religion, disaster, and colonial power in the Spanish Philippines in the sixteenth to seventeenth centuries. *Journal for the Study of Religion, Nature and Culture, 6*, 215–247.

Cannell, F. (1999). *Power and intimacy in the Christian Philippines.* Cambridge University Press.

Constantino, R., & Constantino, L. R. (2008). *A history of the Philippines from the Spanish colonization to the second world war.* NYU Press.

De Bevoise, K. (1995). *Agents of apocalypse: Epidemic disease in the colonial Philippines.* Princeton University Press.

Ileto, R. C. (1979). *Pasyon and revolution: Popular movements in the Philippines, 1840–1910.* Ateneo de Manila University Press.

Ileto, R. C. (1995). *Cholera and the origins of the American sanitary order in the Philippines.* Temple University Press.

Joven, A. E. (2012). Colonial adaptations in tropical Asia: Spanish medicine in the Philippines in the seventeenth and eighteenth centuries. *Asian Cultural Studies, 38*, 171–186.

Junker, L. L. (1999). *Raiding, trading and feasting. The political economy of Philippine Chiefdoms.* University of Hawai'i Press.

Keesing, F. M. (1962). *The ethnohistory of northern Luzon.* Stanford, Calif.: Stanford University Press.

Lynch, O. J. (2011). *Colonial legacies in a fragile republic: A history of Philippine land law and state formation with emphasis on the early U.S. regime (1898–1913).* University of the Philippines, College of Law: U.P. Law Centennial Textbook Project. Philippine Law Collection.

Macdonald, C. J.-H. (2007). *Uncultural behavior, an anthropological investigation of suicide in the southern Philippines.* University of Hawai'i Press.

Mawson, S. (2013). Unruly Plebeians and the Forzado system: Convict transportation between New Spain and the Philippines during the seventeenth century. *Revista de Indias, 73*(259), 693–730. https://doi.org/10.3989/revindias.2013.23

McElhinny, B. (2005). "Kissing a baby is not at all good for him": Infant mortality, medicine, and colonial modernity in the U.S.-occupied Philippines. *American Anthropologist, 107*(2), 183–194.

McNeill, W. H. (1979). *Plagues and peoples*. Penguin.

Mehl, E. M. (2016). *Forced migration in the Spanish Pacific world: From Mexico to the Philippines, 1765–1811 / Eva Maria Mehl*. Cambridge University Press.

Newson, L. A. (1999). Disease and immunity in the pre-Spanish Philippines. *Social Science & Medicine, 48*(12), 1833–1850. ISI://000080764500012.

Pels, P. (1997). The anthropology of colonialism culture, history, and the emergence of western governmentality. http://ezphost.dur.ac.uk/login?url=http://www.jstor.org/stable/2952519

Rafael, V. R. (2018). Colonial contractions: The making of the modern Philippines, 1565–1946. In *Oxford research encyclopedia of Asian history*. Oxford University Press.

Santiago, L. P. R. (1990). The Filipino Indios Encomenderos (ca. 1620–1711). *Philippine Quarterly of Culture and Society, 18*(3), 162–184.

Scalice, J. (2018). Reynaldo Ileto's Pasyon and revolution revisited, a critique. *Sojourn (Singapore), 33*(1), 29. https://doi.org/10.1355/sj33-1b

Smith, W. (2020). *Mountains of blame climate and culpability in the Philippine Uplands / Will Smith*. Seattle University of Washington Press.

Steinberg, D. J. (1990). *The Philippines: A singular and a plural place* (2nd ed.). Westview Press.

Sullivan, R. (1991). Exemplar of Americanism: The Philippine career of Dean C. Worcester.

Tan, S. K. (1987). *A history of the Philippines*. The University of the Philippines Press.

Vallejo, B. (2017). Antonio Luna, science and the emerging Filipino national identity. *Diliman Review, 61*(1).

Warren, J. F. (1981). *The Sulu zone 1768–1898: The dynamics of external trade, slavery, and ethnicity in the transformation of a Southeast Asian Maritime state*. Singapore University Press.

Woods, D. L. (2017). *The myth of the barangay*. University of the Philippines Press.

Worcester, D. C. (1921). *The Philippines past and present* (Vol. 1). Macmillan Company.

3

Practices of Progress

Introduction

In this chapter I focus on the mid-late twentieth-century post-colonial environment in order to contextualise the way in which malaria was implicated in the practices of various professionals who were responsible for directing and delivering health policy in Bataraza in 2012-2014. Following the establishment of the Republic in 1946, Anderson (2007) argues that scientific and biomedical practice was enmeshed in a secular and economic sense of nationalist civic consciousness for a burgeoning elite of Filipinos who increasingly occupied positions within hospitals, universities and research institutes. However, these citizens continued to rely on foreign networks and investment to support their health-related work. As Paterno (2013) argues, the economic, political and health systems of the former colony remained closely modelled on and linked with the United States (US) in particular. Following a period of turbulence, dictatorship and martial law under Ferdinand Marcos, in which scientific research was starved of funds (Anderson, 2007), the People Power Revolution in 1986 ushered in a new political environment of democracy and, with it, an even more aggressive market-orientated economy based on neoliberalism (Paterno, 2013, p. 8). Alongside an upsurge in foreign investment, local government was given unprecedented independence. In terms of malaria, the legacy of these changes was that scientific, biomedical and technological knowledge and practices remained at the heart of contemporary efforts to 'control' and 'eliminate' the disease in official programmes. However, while operationalised on a local level, practices remained tied into a global network of ideas, objectives and, crucially, funders. At the time of my fieldwork, in policy terms at least, the country had moved from trying to 'control' malaria and towards trying to 'eliminate' it, relying heavily on external support, most notably from the Global Fund to Fight AIDS, Tuberculosis and Malaria (GFATM).

It is against this contextual backdrop that I show how contemporary local professionals responsible for designing and implementing health policy in Bataraza enacted a global medical citizenship that continued to be defined relative to an historically contingent transnational web of relations in which malaria initiatives were integrated. As such, I show how for these professionals the adoption of scientific, biomedical and technical knowledge and practices was part of their strategic orientation towards achieving what they described as 'progress' within this interconnected web. Far from simply being imposed from above due to top-down structures of institutional power and uncritically and uniformly accepted, my ethnographic research reveals how these conceptions and practices of malaria were (un)consciously strategically produced and reproduced by health leaders from the bottom up. The reasons behind these enactments being practiced in the arena of formal health policy over others needs to be understood within historical, cultural, political and economic context in order to explain the currency they had (Parker & Allen, 2014). By focussing on how the three main staff responsible for designing and delivering malaria diagnosis and treatment programmes framed and handled malaria in the arena of official programmes, I show how the malaria of progress was cast as a 'top priority' needing investment, something that could be 'cured' through 'compliance' to predominantly biotechnological interventions, and as a knowable disease that Pälawan people could be 'educated' about through biomedically grounded Information Education Campaigns. In spite of some ambiguities, inconsistencies or 'interferences' (Mol, 2002) that existed in this field, these specific ideas and practices were foregrounded over others (through acts of incorporation and distribution) in official programmes as a powerful means for these actors to 'broker' (Nading, 2013; Wolf, 1956) 'progress', both for the Pälawan people they served and for themselves as health leaders in the transnational state.

Malaria Control, Eradication and Elimination in the Post-colonial Period

While the Americans may have signed sovereignty over to the new Philippine state in 1946, independence came hand in hand with continued links to the former ruling nation through the spread of neoliberalist ideas. In terms of economic reform following independence, the US encouraged free trade and, in exchange for the release of war damage payments, required that the constitution be changed to grant US citizens equal rights with Filipino citizens in land ownership, exploitation of natural resources and the operation of public utilities (Paterno, 2013). In 1955, the Laurel Langley Agreement extended liberalised trade further until 1974, perpetuating the neo-colonial nature of the Philippine economy for decades after independence (ibid.). Presidents Elpidio Quirino (1948-1953) and Carlos P. Garcia (1957-1961) managed to boost the countries' economy through more nationalist policies. However, following the authoritarian Marcos regime between 1965 and 1986, which included a period of Martial Law (1972-1986), massive debts were incurred and a neoliberal development paradigm was embraced again by successive administrations to try to enhance the country's economic competitiveness through even more loosened trade and investments, lowered tariffs on imports, wage suppression for global competitiveness, privatisation, reduced government intervention and business deregulation (ibid.). A Structural Adjustment Program imposed by the World Bank meant that in order to continue receiving foreign loans, the country was forced to cut government spending, hitting social services especially hard. In health, this resulted in a reliance on users paying fees alongside a move towards insurance contributory schemes such as PhilHealth. This was accompanied by a steady transition to a devolved system of care. The Department of Health (DOH) was carved out of the colonial Bureau of Public Welfare by the early 1950s (reorganised into the Ministry of Health during the Marcos dictatorship), and the Rural Health Act of 1954 established a nationwide network of Rural Health Units based in the municipalities (towns) and city health centres in the cities. The Local Government Code of 1991 devolved healthcare further giving the DOH jurisdiction only to a provincial level and meaning that provincial, city and municipal government units (LGUs) had significant structural autonomy over care provision (ibid.).

It is within this post-colonial context that the delivery of contemporary malaria 'control' and 'elimination' was shaped in the Philippines and new associations formed between science and biomedicine, healthcare provision and the nature of citizenship. Beyond being implicated in the nationalist movements of the 1940s (Anderson, 2007), Adarlo (2017) demonstrates how even more recently the promotion of science and technology education was key to fostering a sense of national identity, following the post-martial law government and the re-writing of the constitution in 1987. The uptake and promotion of science and technology that continued among health policy staff at the time of my fieldwork must therefore be understood against this backdrop. Together, this combination of factors shaped the formation and aims of various malaria policies which local actors enabled and enacted. Many have documented how rhetoric around malaria in medicine, academia, politics and philanthropy remains infused with military metaphor to describe both malaria and the attempts to deal with it, particularly following World War II (Brown, 1997; Brown & Inhorn, 1997; Kelly & Beisel, 2011). I too have suggested elsewhere that a combination of the failure of early post-war eradication campaigns and the reduction in global malaria rates over the last decade in particular have resulted in changes to the semantic field which has now taken on a more nuanced and positive tone, speaking instead of 'control' and referring to concepts such as 'sustaining the gains', 'making durable progress', 'shrinking the malaria map', 'maintaining progress' and so on (Iskander, 2015). Malaria is nevertheless cast as an object of 'monitoring', 'surveillance' 'control' or even 'eradication' using a complicated mix of standardised technical solutions (Chandler et al., 2014). This is mirrored in national- and local-level policy discourse and practice in the Philippines.

In terms of country-specific malaria-related strategy, comprehensive accounts are provided by Russell (1936), Ejercito et al. (1954) and a more recent co-authored report by the Ministry of Health Philippines et al. (2014). To summarise, a National Malaria Control Programme (NMCP) was adopted in 1902 and 'control' was formally undertaken by the American administration through a combination of administering mosquito nets for prevention (although mainly to the US army) and the drug quinine for treatment. Freshwater mosquitofish (Gambusia) were also introduced to Manila in 1913 from Texas in order to feed on mosquito larvae in certain locations as a form of biological control. The Americans reorganised the Bureau of Public Welfare and oversaw the establishment of the Philippine Health Service (PHS) (a precursor to the Department of Health) with support from the International Health Division of the Rockefeller Foundation. The PHS were charged with carrying out centralised malaria surveillance and the Malaria Control Section and the Advisory Committee for Malaria Control were later established to institute preventive measures and treatment protocols. After World War II, and the formation of the WHO in 1948, malaria was high on the international agenda, affecting as it did many countries touched by war. In post-war Philippines, under a newly forming Republic, malaria-related activities remained centralised and bolstered by the US PHS but now operated through the Philippine Health Rehabilitation Programme (PHRR) that had stalled in the war years, contributing to a steady rise in malaria cases. Under the PHRR, the Malaria Division was responsible for decision-making as well as administrative and technical oversight of a number of biotechnological interventions to help control the disease. Provincial hospitals began keeping malaria surveillance records and conducting microscopic examinations, treating cases with the drugs quinine or chloroquine as recommended by the WHO. These methods were used alongside the distribution of mosquito screens and nets for use in homes and some environmental measures including the drainage of breeding sites and the use of Paris Green (an arsenic-based larvicide) at breeding sites. In 1948, DDT (dicophane pesticide) was also used by the US PHS on a small scale for spraying houses, with a larger programme sponsored by the WHO taking place between 1952 and 1954 in Mindoro province. Together, these interventions resulted in a substantial decline in malaria morbidity by 1955 and 'control' began to shift towards 'eradication' (Ministry of Health Philippines et al., 2014).

The change in strategy towards 'eradication' mirrored global agendas and rhetoric and relied yet again on external support, mainly from the WHO and the United States Agency for International Development (USAID). As Packard (1997) explains, the WHO-led worldwide eradication campaign 'both reflected and was part of this growing faith in the ability of western science and technology to transform underdeveloped countries. This faith was part of what has been called the "culture of development". The attitude of "know how and show how" [that] emerged out of the War' (ibid., p. 288). In 1956, the Philippine Congress passed the Malaria Eradication Bill and the Joint Philippine-American Malaria Eradication Programme was implemented from 1956 to 1960 (Ministry of Health Philippines et al., 2014). The aim was to develop a curriculum that the Philippine government could take over and maintain until eradication was achieved. Attempts to eradicate in the 1950s coincided with some early efforts to devolve care. The Department of Health was restructured in 1959 under the Reorganisation Act and delegated responsibility of malaria-related activities to regional personnel. However, poor implementation led to an increase in annual incidence of malaria between 1960 and 1965 and eventual recentralisation in 1966 (Espino et al., 2004). When external support from USAID was withdrawn in 1973 the government was unable to sustain its programmes and many were abandoned. Political unrest and population movement contributed to an increase in cases and eradication was officially left behind in 1983, again mirroring policy shifts elsewhere that acknowledged that the worldwide eradication of the diseases was not going to be possible (Ministry of Health Philippines et al., 2014).

A move back towards 'control' in the 1980s came with increasing devolution. In 1979, the Philippines had signed up to the Alma Ata Declaration, which 'provided a manifesto for mass access to healthcare that linked poor health with poverty, and proposed responses that moved away from relying on largely biomedical solutions to reactively lessen the burden of ill-health' (Parker & Allen, 2014, p. 226). Instead, 'Primary

Health Care and Health for All by 2000' became national policy (Paterno, 2013) with a focus on more preventative, holistic and localised approaches. Accordingly, responsibility for implementing healthcare was transferred to LGUs in 1991. This shifted oversight and functions (services, personnel, assets and liabilities) of all health, education, agriculture and social service to cities, provinces and municipalities and was aimed at 'empowering' LGUs to approach health as an integrated and local issue (ibid.). In this devolved structure, the DOH served as the lead governing agency with both local LGUs and the private sectors providing services to the population on the ground (Paterno, 2013). However, as Espino et al. (2004) document, the 'semi-vertical' nature of the health system was problematic as municipal malaria coordinators were theoretically responsible for implementing programme operations with little funding from local governments. Instead, they had to rely again on international funding in addition to the private sector. In the 1990s, malaria initiatives were therefore mainly funded by the World Bank via the Philippine Health Development Project which allocated 6% of its overall US $68.2 million budget to malaria-related interventions, namely vector control using insecticides and case detection (Ministry of Health Philippines et al., 2014). To a large extent, devolution in the 1980s and 1990s was poorly implemented (Bossert et al., 2000) and resulted in a fragmentation of administrative services between hospitals and RHUs; confusion over who was mandated with specific responsibilities; and limited improvement in actual service delivery (Bossert et al., 2000; Espino et al., 2004). Following a surge of malaria cases in the 1980s, the urgent objective was to reverse the trend and address the challenges of devolution (Ministry of Health Philippines et al., 2014).

Malaria 'control' efforts towards the end of the century did eventually successfully result in a reduction of cases to the extent that in November 1997, after a year of intensive local and national consultation, a malaria 'elimination' strategy was launched with the goal of achieving a malaria-free Philippines by 2020. As the country entered this new phase, the health sector was reformed yet again, promoting the development of even more localised health systems and improving domestic financing (Romualdez Jr et al., 2011). Strengthened local ownership was coupled with a substantial increase in external funding from sources such as

Department of Foreign Affairs and Trade of Australia (DFAT), the WHO-Roll Back Malaria (WHO-RBM) initiative and, mainly, from the GFATM, leading to a massive scale-up in malaria-related interventions and activities. These additional resources augmented the yearly allocation to LGUs from the national budget. This sets the scene for malaria-related policies, firmly orientated towards 'elimination' at the time of my field-work. What became apparent through examination of the history of malaria control, eradication and elimination efforts in the post-colonial period is that local health actors continued to operate in similar global networks that shaped their strategic aims, practices and the very malaria that was enacted as a result.

Eliminating Malaria in Bataraza: Practices of Progress

In Bataraza, for health leaders charged with implementing malaria-related policy, 'elimination' was at the forefront of everyone's mind. In 2007, the DOH launched the disease-elimination zone initiative, setting aside specific funds (169 million Pesos/US $3.8 million) for this purpose (DOH, 2011). In 2009, the Philippines joined the Asia Pacific Malaria Elimination Network (APMEN) and the most recent Malaria Medium Term Development Plan (2011–2016) from the DOH reiterated the aim of achieving a Malaria-Free Philippines. Here, I describe how the practices of the Medical Health Technician (MHT), the Municipal Health Officer (MHO) and the Community Relation Officer (CRO) were orientated towards achieving what they described as different kinds of 'progress' in line with their positions as 'global medical citizens' in the field of official malaria programmes. Within anthropological scholarship, medical citizenship (also referred to as biological citizenship, biocitizenship or health citizenship) has been used to describe various ways in which health becomes intertwined with citizens' sense of subjectivity, belonging and their rights and responsibilities within a nation. Health becomes an arena through which citizens are thus able to negotiate the provision of health-care, access to it and social, political and economic inclusion for others more broadly (Biehl, 2004; Fassin, 2009; Nguyen, 2010; Petryna, 2013; Rose, 2007; Rose & Novas, 2005). Specifically, I follow Nading (2013) in arguing that health leaders enacted a dual form of medical citizenship that put them in a conflicted position and created a collision of interests (Wolf, 1956). On the one hand, they acted as agents of the state, tasked with achieving 'progress' in the form of meeting targets, securing funding and investment and implementing healthcare more broadly in line with national and transnational directives. On the other, they acted as representatives of and advocates for 'progress' on behalf of the local people for whom they cared—namely Pälawan communities amongst whom malaria rates were highest. As 'brokers' (ibid.) between global organisations and the state as well as citizens, their (un)conscious strategic aim was to 'master' (Bourdieu, 1977) progress for both in the field of official healthcare provision. However, in so doing, they implicated a certain kind of malaria alongside their practices—one that was a 'top priority', could be 'cured' with biotechnological interventions and one that could be communicated about using biomedical education campaigns. Whilst of benefit to Pälawan citizens to some extent, enacting malaria in this way also had its costs for local communities that leaders were all too aware of as I go on to describe.

A 'Top Priority'

I sit on a wooden stool just outside Maria's office in the RHU. She is wearing a t-shirt with the statement '*Kilusang Ligtas Malaria*' (Movement Against Malaria) emblazoned on it and her office walls were adorned with posters related to malaria as well as charts where she records the number of microscopic tests she performs every day. I watch her carry out her work as I have done many times before. On her bench is her microscope, slides boxes, stains and piles of folders and paperwork. On a metal trolly outside the office door is a box of disposable gloves, small squares of gauze, balls of cotton wool soaked in alcohol, glass slides, blood lancets and a stack of paper slips. She summons the lady sitting next to me to her as she stands at the trolly. She gently takes her finger in her gloved hand as they talk about the impending rain, rubs her finger clean with a ball of cotton wool and massages it to stimulate blood flow. She pricks the side of her fingertip with a lancet which she discards into a small yellow waste box on the floor. As a drop of blood appears on the edge of the lady's finger, Maria applies a slide to it to transfer drops of blood onto the glass. She uses another piece of glass to spread out the blood spots, one is so thinly smeared across the bottom half of the slide, I can hardly see it, while a larger drop at the top is spread more thickly. She places the labelled slide into the slide box on her desk and tells the lady to wait for the result. 'Have you had any positive cases today?' I ask her. 'No', she replies. 'Like every day, most will be negative for malaria'. Just then, Danny appears. Him and Maria are about to go to their regular meeting with the other microscopists from each of the 22 *Barangay* Health Stations dotted around the municipality as they do every Monday. He looks a little stressed. He picks up a folder from the desk and looks through the slips of paper that correspond to the slides him and Maria have tested that week. 'Ah, there was one positive last week. Did they return for their follow-up smear?.' Maria replies that the patient did and their smear was negative, pointing to another slip in the folder. 'That's good right?' I say. Danny replies 'Yes, but even to have one case of malaria here is bad. We will have to see how many other positive cases the microscopists found but already this is a bad start to the week for me. Let's see what happens at our meeting.'

Since devolution, implementation of the National Malaria Control Programme was semi-vertical as described earlier; meaning malaria surveillance, treatment and diagnosis was carried out on a local level through the RHU where Maria and Danny were stationed. The DOH set overall policies, targets and standards. In addition, they provided technical training and quality assurance for diagnosis, treatment and vector control measures; designed health promotion materials; augmented the logistical requirements of LGUs; and conducted regular monitoring and evaluation across the country. In Palawan, as in other provinces, the DOH operated though a Provincial Health Office (PHO) where DOH representatives were positioned (Liu et al., 2013). PHOs provided information, training and technical assistance to each municipality and to staff such as Danny, the Coordinator of vector-borne diseases and Medical Technician, who was responsible for the day-to-day implementation and delivery of malaria-related surveillance, diagnostic and treatment services. In Bataraza, in addition to Danny and the microscopist, Maria, the RHU housed the only doctor or Municipal Health Officer (MHO), one dentist, two nurses and two midwives. Each of the 22 *barangays* had their own *Barangay* Health Station (BHS) which in turn employed midwives, sanitary inspectors, nutritional specialists and microscopists (usually one to two of each). In addition, each BHS also had a number of voluntary *Barangay* Health Workers (BHWs) who operated within the community and, as such, played an instrumental role in providing primary healthcare to the population in areas such as infectious disease, hygiene and sanitation and maternal, new-born and child health. In some *barangays*, one BHW was also trained as a specialist in carrying out malaria Rapid Diagnostic Tests (RDTs) which were portable, gave results in minutes and could be deployed in people's homes with ease. In Bataraza, there was one private hospital in the *barangay* of Rio Tuba which was established by the Rio Tuba Nickel Foundation as part of their corporate social responsibility activities and it provided free healthcare only to some in the municipality that lived closest to it. The nearest government hospital where free treatment was available to all was in the neighbouring municipality of Brooke's Point. As such, the government-run RHU and its staff were the main providers of free primary care within Bataraza. In this setting, malaria monitoring, diagnosis and treatment was part of the day-to-day practice of health staff. In fact, it was the centre of much of their rhetoric and practice.

For Danny, even one positive case of malaria was 'bad' because he, like all health leaders in the Bataraza, was aiming to eliminate the disease completely from the islands. In a devolved system, the pressure was therefore on him to achieve results. As he explained:

I have been the Coordinator of malaria activities here in Bataraza since 2004. In that time, positive cases in the whole municipality have been just over 1,000 each year which is considered high compared to other parts of the country. We had a major epidemic in 2004 and then again in 2006 when cases went up to almost 1,700. But we have had only one death here in the time I have been here in 2008. A man died only a few hours after he had received a positive smear test. He had delayed treatment because he had gone to the *balyan* (healer) who did not diagnose malaria so it was already too late for him. Apart from this one, there has been no mortality due to malaria. Cases actually dropped again until 2010, when we had another outbreak because our monitoring was lower in that year and we only did one round of house spraying because of limited funding. Last year [2012], we were very high in terms of cases again in the whole of the province and this year [2013], sad to say we came back up to first place. In 2011, we actually had only 694 cases reported from all the *Barangay* Health Stations. It isn't that high compared to other diseases. But even this it is not good enough. Our target is to be malaria-free by 2020 and so malaria is really our top priority. It is my duty to make sure we do that and that our activities and staff have the necessary funding to do what they need to do to prevent all malaria here. It isn't just the Philippines that is trying to eliminate malaria, many countries can now do this and it is a global target. There is a lot of pressure on me to reach the target but our problem is we are so dependent on what comes from international sources so we do not always have the means to progress in this goal.

In 2012, when I began fieldwork, only around 20% of the population of the Philippines were living in malaria-free areas (i.e., zero Indigenous cases). As Danny intimated, places such as Palawan had high transmission particularly in areas such as Bataraza. Danny had clearly overseen some success in lowering rates over the last decade, but in reality, continued transmission in areas such as his meant formal targets set by the NMCP had actually dropped the stipulation to eliminate malaria by 2020. In fact, in 2012 the WHO declared that the Philippines was 'officially' classified as in the 'control' phase (ibid., p. 57). Nevertheless, 'elimination' was the goal that Danny, and all the formal health leaders and workers I spoke to articulated as what they were working towards. As he put it, it was his 'duty' to achieve 'progress' in this goal—pulling him into not only national but global agendas. Alongside Danny, a major player in building and maintaining support for malaria-related activities, communicating developments and securing investment at a local government level was the MHO, Reyna. The MHO was technically responsible for briefing political figures on health matters and formulating policies at the municipal level that conform to national and international policies (Espino et al., 2004). Reyna was coming to the end of her two-year deployment to the municipality as part of the 'Doctor to the Barrios[1]' scheme, established by the DOH in 1993. This incentive-based placement programme recruited newly graduated medical doctors for redeployment in rural, geographically isolated and underserved municipalities (Avanceña et al., 2019). Renya was regularly away from the RHU, conducting medical 'missions' or taking part in career development training. In her absence, Danny was therefore often left as acting-MHO and, in reality, the person largely responsible for delivering and managing malaria programmes on the ground. Both Danny and Renya told me that despite having a number of other responsibilities, malaria took up the vast majority of their time and effort. It was something that they both described as their 'priority'. As Renya articulated, 'most malaria cases are among the most vulnerable in our municipality, the IPs [Indigenous Peoples]—so it is our major priority to do what we can in malaria above all else to help them and have no cases here in Bataraza'. In meetings that I attended in the RHU, led by Danny or Renya, malaria was always first on the list for discussion and often described in this way. However, as alluded to above by Maria, while cases may have been relatively high compared to the rest of the country and therefore an obstacle to national and international goals, in absolute terms they were rather low, especially compared to cases of other diseases as discussed below. This was the paradox that surrounded malaria in Bataraza. I encountered it in many fields and among many players, not just among health leaders. The disease was simultaneously the focus of so much attention, both rhetorical and practical, at the same time as it posed a relatively trivial threat to people's health and wellbeing compared to other health and social issues. For health leaders, eliminating malaria was their 'top priority' but making progress was about much more than purging parasites.

For actors such as Danny and Renya, the prioritisation of malaria was driven less by the presence of pathogenic organisms and more by the structure of health financing on which they were 'so dependent' as Danny stated. It was his responsibility to compile malaria rates from across the municipality in his Monday meetings as well as compute expenditure on

---

[1] In Spanish, *barrio* translates into English as 'quarter'. In the Philippines it is used to denote a rural village.

malaria-related activities in order to request funding from the PHO and the Local Health Board which, in turn, advised the municipal council regarding its allocations for public health activities. As Danny explained, this investment was crucial beyond just its implications for malaria:

> Money from the Global Fund [GFATM] provides 80% of the budget for malaria and is … [for] drugs, nets, the salary of the spray men, RDT supplies and most important some of the salary incentives of health workers from the PHO. The other 20% of the budget comes from the municipality and is for incentives for microscopists and their lab supplies, gloves, slides. But no [laughs], in the future, I do not think we will have enough money to support all this once the Global Fund money ends. That is our problem. This money is for malaria but it supports all our system in reality—our staff incentives and our general supplies. I don't know what we will do when it ends. … I am worried. … We are in the transition period now … so what we are doing is the allocations … of the commodities that the Global Fund has given to us until 2014. If we can supplement this from the LGU and from the PHO then it's ok. So, we are doing our best now to gain [their] support. … Hopefully there will be another funding programme from the Global Fund that can renew the money because we don't have any idea now if they will continue the funding or stop it in 2014. What we know here is that the Global Fund money will end in 2014 but there are some meetings at the upper level and they are still trying to convince [them] to continue their support for Tuberculosis, malaria and HIV. … It is up to me to show we can make progress to eliminate malaria so that we can have enough money to continue all our other work here. We need to pay our own salaries but also those of other staff and to secure all the programmes that we need. I see this as one of my main responsibilities.

As described above, current funding and delivery of malaria services was shared between the national and local governments and private health providers but to a large extent still depended on international agencies, namely the GFATM. GFATM support in the Philippines began in 2002 when US $40 million was awarded to two non-profit organisations—the Tropical Disease Foundation and the Pilipinas Shell Foundation, Inc (PSFI) (the social arm of Shell companies in the Philippines). Subsequent funding was awarded, and by 2010, all existing

GFATM malaria grants were consolidated into a single one covering 40 malaria-endemic provinces including Palawan (UCSF, 2012). At the time of fieldwork, total malaria-specific funding for the country had reached over US $82 million meaning the Philippines was still hugely reliant on funding from external sources. This was particularly significant as the GFATM investment was possibly going to come to an end in 2014 because of revised grant allocation criteria as Danny suggested, leaving the burden of financing future activities and healthcare more generally to the government. In Palawan, PSFI had worked in cooperation with Kilusan Ligtas Malaria (KLM) (Movement Against Malaria) since 1999, who, along with the PHO, implemented malaria programmes across the Island. As Danny explained, in Bataraza, financial support from PSFI/KLM through the PHO made up the vast majority of the total spend on malaria activities. Only a minority was met by the municipal and *barangay* allocations. At the time, the Philippines lacked a long-term, sustainable domestic strategy to finance activities such as IRS and net distribution as well as support staff positions in the 40 provinces supported by the GFATM (UCSF, 2012). Government data suggested that domestic malaria funding was targeted only towards the malaria-free provinces, leaving the current GFATM-supported provinces which had active transmission such as Palawan at real risk of disinvestment and subsequent resurgence once this funding source ended. This situation made the uncertainty about the continuation of international grants a real worry for Danny. He was caught in a double bind of at once having to demonstrate success in eliminating malaria to international organisations in order to justify current investment whilst simultaneously running the risk that his very success in doing so could lead to a reduction in their main sources of financial support in the future.

In addition to being tied into fiscal incentives, meeting the target of elimination and securing investment was also caught up in the career development and satisfaction of health leaders such as Renya who explains:

> For me, this is what I feel I can achieve in this posting. I wanted to come to a rural place like this because it is my passion to serve the people here, especially the IPs. This is why I became a doctor after all. So, to prove to

my superiors I have done a good job here, we must also eliminate malaria, despite all the challenges we face trying to do that. I do not know if it will be possible to but I want my time here in the provinces to be successful for myself too. That is why all of us must work so hard, Danny and I especially. It is our responsibility to make sure this happens—it is our job to improve the health of the people here. That is how we will know we have done well in our own careers.

Similar feelings were expressed by health staff lower down the chain of command—the BHWs, for whom malaria was also articulated as a 'top priority', both in terms of caring for their patients and in terms of caring about their careers. This was despite the fact that many BHWs, similar to Renya, were dubious about the possibility of realising the goal in actuality. Ramil once said to me, in reference to his wife Babydan's work at an RDT specialist:

> In the RHU or even the BHSs, if they see even one case of malaria then they will get disappointed. Even my wife, because of the command of her superior, she is also so upset when people arrive in the house and get [one] positive [result] for malaria then she is disappointed. They are very determined to be successful in their jobs and make zero malaria both for the people and for themselves.

As such, while malaria was implicated in health leaders' genuine compassionate desire to ensure the good health of people in their community, it was also embroiled in their (un)conscious efforts to secure wider investment in health services from a range of national and international actors and ensure success in their own careers. Prioritising malaria through rhetoric and practice did not occur so much *in response* to parasites; after all, there were not that many circulating around the population. Rather, malaria was enacted as a 'top priority' alongside a series of other strategically orientated practices aimed at achieving 'progress' of different guises more generally in the field of local health policy.

However, this focus on malaria also came at a price for Pälawan communities. Having lived in upland areas to carry out medical missions or to act as gatekeeper and research assistant for various health and livelihood projects, Danny, in particular, was very aware of what he described as many more 'urgent' health problems. He often told me that poverty was a much more pressing issue for the people he served, as well as basic hygiene and sanitation. As a result, it was not surprising to him that the rates of infectious diseases such as diarrhoea, cholera and tuberculosis were much higher among the Pälawan than malaria in his monthly surveillance reports. Accordingly, he acknowledged the 'over-emphasis' that was put on malaria and told me that this was in some ways at odds with his 'duty' to help people with the health issues that most afflicted them. When I asked Ramil if a similar focus was put on other health issues his answer was that 'generally speaking, no. There is a, how shall [I] say, [an] *out* of focus. Other kinds of diseases are out of focus.' This view was also shared by Renya:

> The biggest problem here among the IPs is diarrhoea and hygiene. They live in very remote places without even electricity, running water or toilets and for many of them work is difficult to find for money. Tuberculosis is also a big problem and we had a very serious Cholera epidemic last year. Malaria is not such a big problem for them because it is treatable and preventable and all the people here know about it so is not the priority in some ways. But it is the thing that receives the most focus. We are trying to do our best to help them as much as we can—this is why I came here to this remote place. It is a hard place to be because there are so many problems but it is my mission. These people need our help with many issues, not just malaria, but with their situations in life, but in a way, malaria can also be a way to do these other things.

For Renya and Danny, despite being aware of other more pressing health concerns for Pälawan people in Bataraza, this contestation or 'interference', as Mol (2002) calls it, was actively harnessed in such a way as to bolster, rather than undermine, the prioritisation of malaria for them. The legitimate deprioritisation of malaria among Pälawan communities was acknowledged, but gave these particular health professionals even more impetus to take up the mantle of highlighting it in governance arenas as a route to helping them carry out other strategic aims including dealing with the other health and social concerns of the Pälawan. The divergence remained but sat next to, assembled alongside and was even incorporated into the prioritised malaria that leaders enacted in order to fulfil their aims. In this way, malaria as both priority and posteriority were made to be mutually inclusive (Strathern, 1991). Practically and rhetorically framing malaria as a 'top priority' enabled Danny and Renya to garner social, professional, economic and political power in their field. It was a means for them to enact their 'responsibility', duty' and 'mission' as global medical citizens, enmeshed as they were in a web of international, national and local relationships, both for themselves and for the people they served. As Renya alluded to above, making 'progress' in this field also entailed framing and enacting malaria as a preventable and treatable disease—one that could be 'cured' through a series of biotechnological interventions, despite the interferences that were implicated in this approach too.

A 'Curable' Disease

In terms of the methods promoted to 'control' and 'eliminate' malaria through the NMCP, 'a biomedical model' pervaded. However, as the WHO and DOH make explicit, there was acknowledgement that on the ground at least, these framings and practices existed alongside a plurality of systems and models:

> Health service delivery is based on a Western biomedical model of health initially introduced during the Spanish colonial era and strengthened during American colonization. This Western system is superimposed on a pre-existing alternative model of health care based on a mix of folk and herbal medicines, religious beliefs, and traditional practices that has persisted throughout the country. (WHO/DOH, 2012)

In Bataraza, it was clear that health leaders similarly acknowledged a range of possible ways citizens understood and dealt with malaria, as is discussed in more detail below. However, in official programmes, Danny and Renya nevertheless framed and enacted a kind of malaria that, as well as being a priority, could be 'monitored', 'prevented' and 'treated' using a set of internationally recognised, standardised biotechnological interventions. As Danny explained:

Cases have certainly dropped directly because of what we are doing here. Since I have been the Coordinator, the trend for the malaria positivity cases is between March to June before the really heavy rain starts so all of our preventive measures against the vectors are done in December to March in preparation for peak season. Monitoring and surveillance is very important. Each month we record the number of cases and stratify the *sitios* [units or villages within *barangays*] based on where we find one case. Each BHS records the cases from microscopy and the RDT specialists if they have one. This is very important so that we know where exactly to target our efforts. For example, now we are again starting our IRS spraying that happens twice a year in February and August. We only do IRS in malarious areas where there is at least one case from the monitoring. Every house [in that area] will have it done twice in the year. Bed nets are also redistributed twice a year for free in all areas regardless of whether or not there are cases. We have been doing that since 2004. We are also doing our distribution again now too. Long-lasting nets are better because they don't need to be dipped so we give those now and it is a lot easier. We do twice a year because some families are newly arrived or just married and may not have one for their own household. We give only to ones who need it so we only replace nets which are dilapidated. On the side of people, we are also doing our Information Education Campaigns (IECs). So, there is a lot we do to prevent malaria.

Similarly, when it came to diagnosis and treatment, PSFI/KLM through the PHO funded microscopists such as Maria in all *barangays* as well as a limited number of RDT specialists such as Babydan in *barangays* that had the highest rates of malaria. There were eight trained RDT personnel in the whole municipality at the time I was there. All anti-malarial drugs were provided for free at the point of care and funded by the GFATM through PSFI/KLM. As Renya suggested, it was through these interventions that they hoped to 'cure' people of the disease stating, 'Malaria is a 100% curable disease. We follow the WHO guidelines and have drugs like Coartem[2] for *falciparum* and Chloroquine for *vivax*. That is how we will reach our target of elimination. Through nets, spraying, testing, drugs we can do it.'

It was no surprise that Danny and Renya framed and enacted malaria in line with scientific and biomedical traditions. Both were trained in government institutions in Manila in medical technology and medicine respectively. As such, they mobilised a similar set of theoretical frameworks, techniques and instruments in order to design and implement policies and meet targets that had been set by institutions that based healthcare delivery on the same models. It was also with recourse to these frameworks that these actors lobbied local government leaders in the discussions that I observed. Geographical areas were mapped, stratified and labelled as 'risky'; figures, charts and tables of cases were quantified and presented; materials and supplies were accounted for; and budgets were justified, estimated and requested. However, alongside these framings and enactments, as before, there was also 'interference'. As practised health professionals, both Danny and Renya had direct experience trying to decipher and implement these seemingly neutral ways of viewing malaria, the environment it existed in and the biotechnological interventions designed to deal with it in real-world situations where they encountered a number of 'difficulties. This was clear in many conversations I had with Danny such as this:

Malaria is really a significant problem in those areas because of the attitude of most of our IPs [Indigenous Peoples]. They are the ones who are really affected but we have many difficulties in identifying and treating all the cases. We still cannot change their practices and beliefs towards the treatment and compliance of malaria and the compliance of using bed nets and the IRS [Indoor Residual Spraying]. In reality, we have a lot of difficulties with these measures in these communities. For example, the IPs are not so interested in malaria that's the first thing. They have other concerns about daily life. Also, because of their culture they are more at risk. For example, they sit out at night and watch videos on Betamax because this is their only entertainment and expose themselves to the mosquitoes. When I stay with

---

[2] Coartem is the company Novartis' brand name for their artemether-lumefantrine combination anti-malarial drug.

them, even myself, I do this. With the drugs, because of the Education Campaigns, they know about *falciparum* malaria so even when they come here to the clinic they say they have *falciparum*—they know about it—but then they take Chloroquine—they take it for everything even though now it is only recommended for *vivax* because it is cheap and they can buy it themselves in the *sari-sari* (road-side variety store). They can buy just one or two tablets. It is cheaper for them to do that than come here to the RHU to get the right drugs for free. Compliance is our biggest problem, you know like hoarding of drugs—it is their culture to keep them in their roof or they take the it only until symptoms get better and then keep the rest for next time to save their money. They have very little money. … Some people don't use their nets for sleeping but use them for fishing once they have a hole in them. For them, fishing is very important for their livelihood to have food and even sell for money. I have seen that. We are also having problems with them being nomadic as they tend to transfer from one place to another. When they do their *kaingin* (Tagalog for swidden), they camp in temporary places and don't use any nets. Maybe that is why rates our higher in summer too, because it is so hot and they don't take nets up there. Even in the very far *barangays,* if they need to see the doctor, they will bring their whole family—that is also part of their culture, to always be together. They have motorcycles with supports on each side so that eight or nine people can ride on one motor but that is why they don't come because there are so many of them and the fare is high or they cannot afford the gasoline for all those people. … So, I think we could not eradicate malaria because of them. That's our problem.

In Danny's description of the issues implementing biotechnological interventions in Pälawan communities, a whole host of practices and relations were lumped together under the category of 'cultural' impediments to 'compliance'. These ranged from watching Betamax videos to being too poor to afford access to formal healthcare. Structural complexes were translated into individual-level 'cultural' 'risk factors' and pitted against neutral interventions. Day-to-day, health leaders invested a considerable amount of time in trying to ensure 'compliance' and in this way enacted a medical citizenship that was also top-down, disciplinary and bureaucratic as much as it was localised, compassionate and flexible (Nading, 2013).

Renya too told me that her experience of working in Bataraza conformed her view that, ultimately, issues relating to health extended beyond discrete biomedical models of disease that decontextualised causation, prevention and treatment. However, she acknowledged that dealing with these more social and relational factors lay outside of her capacity and remit as a doctor:

> At the end of the day, what I have realised is that if you improve poverty and living standards, malaria will go away and health will improve in general for these people. It is all related. You cannot expect people to be able to improve malaria alone without these other things that affect daily life being understood and dealt with but I cannot do this as a doctor. All I can do is diagnose and treat malaria with what I am given and tell people to comply.

As a result, in order to deal with these complexities, interferences were distributed into the domain of 'culture' by health leaders who were unable to 'tackle' them under the rubric of 'health'. While they had biotechnological interventions to approach disease (as a natural discrete entity) at their disposal, they did not have the structural tools needed to 'tackle' the messiness and particularity of 'culture'. As Blaser (2018) explains distribution works by 'keeping different performances apart so that inconsistencies between them do not turn into clashes where some sort of adjudication of "truth" has to occur to preserve the unity of a given object' (ibid., p. 51). By strategically enacting malaria as a discrete, natural phenomenon that could be cured with universally applicable biotechnological interventions in the domain of health, health leaders such as Danny and Renya were able to make 'progress'. Danny articulated this directly when he told me: 'We cannot eradicate poverty here and solve all the social issues. We cannot change the culture of the people. All we can do is make programmes to help prevent disease as best we can. Malaria, we can make progress with through all we are doing. Maybe the rest will follow. That is my hope.' As described in the next section, one of the primary ways that health leaders tried to achieve 'progress' for their citizens and 'compliance' to biotechnological solutions was through mass education campaigns.

A 'Knowable' Disease

I asked Michael what the biggest obstacles he faced in his job were. He replied, that in terms of 'barriers to elimination, well wrong information. Because sometimes the IPs [Indigenous Peoples], the beliefs that they inherited from their ancestors are still intact. Like when you drink coconut water you will get malaria. And the 'quack' doctors. When the person gets sick even when you teach them to go to the Health Centre right away, they still go to the 'quack' doctor because they believe he can cure them because they believe if they have a fever, it is not malaria but something called *bati*[3]. ... Even when I will conduct IECs [Information Education Campaigns] they don't listen. If you go there, they say "yes we understand" and then when we come back again, they say "no we don't' do that still" and we must start again in educating them' I was taking to Michael as we prepared slides together sitting under a tree for shade. I had met Danny, Michael and the other staff from the RHU very early in the morning in order to help them conduct the day's scheduled 'medical mission'. To get to our destination, we took the only ambulance the RHU had to the shore, from where we took a boat across as the *sitio* we were heading to was best accessible by water. The ambulance was old, shabby and dirty with only a stretcher and stethoscope inside. We loaded it with 200 or so Long-Lasting Insecticide Nets alongside other boxes of supplies including equipment to take blood smears to test for malaria. After the hour-long boat ride, we arrived on the other side and loaded carabao-driven (water buffalo) ploughs with our boxes. The animals pushed on ahead as we walked barefoot across muddy mangroves for around 40 minutes. When we arrived at the school building, we washed out feet under a water pump, donned our flipflops, drank hot coffee from thermos flasks and waited under a tree for people to arrive. By midday, a large crowd of men, women and children had gathered. One BHW was conducting screening for Tuberculosis while the midwife gave out Vitamin A tablets to pregnant women and the dentist checked people's teeth, giving out toothbrushes as she did so. Michael, the Community Relation Officer, set up table and chairs in the shade for us. I helped him keep the slides in order as he took people's blood, transferring

---

[3] *Bati* comes from *nabati* in Tagalog meaning to be greeted, or *salibegbeg/samban* in Palawano, and refers to sicknesses presenting as fever, chilling, sweating, body pain, rashes, insomnia and the body becoming 'stiff' or 'too strong' to move. *Bati/salibegbeg* comes about due to angered *diwata* (spirits) speaking the name of the aggressor or brushing past them resulting in misfortune or illness.

spots onto slides that I labelled and filed, which would be screened for malaria. Danny meanwhile, distributed bed nets, ticking off and updating recipients' names on a list he had of the inhabitants of the 160 or so households. The last time they distributed bed nets was almost six years ago and many people brought their old damaged nets to show Danny, explaining how the holes meant mosquitoes could get through despite their best efforts to repair them. … A couple of hours passed. Danny and Michael rounded the children up into one of the classrooms to conduct an IEC. They had written the symptoms of various fever-related illnesses on the board and were going through them individually. They started with malaria. 'If you get a fever' Michael said 'you should immediately tell your mother or father to take you to the Health Centre and get a smear test for malaria. If you have *falciparum*, you need to take Coartem and this will be given to you for free. You should only take Chloroquine if you have *vivax* malaria. That is why you need to have a test—to find out which kind of malaria you have.' He explained how malaria parasites were spread to people by mosquitos and when peak biting times were (between 6pm and 6am). Danny took over, telling the children how they could help prevent malaria by draining stagnant water where mosquitos bred in rubbish and coconut shells, by keeping carabao close to the house so that mosquitos would bite them rather than people and showing them how to use and care for their new bed nets. They were both animated and made the session participative by teaching the children a song, in which they pretended to be buzzing mosquitoes, showing the audience how to slap mosquitoes off their skin. The children were laughing, singing and shouting back answers to the quiz questions Michael asked at the end. Him and Danny continued talking about the other diseases on the board—Dengue, Typhoid, Tuberculosis and Urinary Tract Infections. No more songs were sung and the performance got a little less animated as time went on. In truth, I started to switch off and took the opportunity to write up my fieldnotes instead. The heat and tiredness of the day caught up with me and my concentration was slipping as I slowly got confused about the differences between all the causes, symptoms, treatments and preventative measures they were talking about for various febrile illnesses. The next day, it was malaria that had stuck in my mind and I was sure it would have been the same for the children.

As described above, funding from PSFI/KLM included the provision of a Community Relation Officer (CRO) in Bataraza—Michael. His principal function was to hold regular IECs within communities that had reported at least one malaria case in the previous month. Michael therefore worked in close collaboration with the Danny and they often conducted IECs together, combining malaria-specific activities such as screening, net distribution and education events with wider 'medical missions' as described above. Danny and his team at the RHU also broadcast a weekly radio programme on the local station and their voices regularly floated over the airwaves, even in the most secluded corners of the municipality. Like Danny, Michael was friendly, outgoing and charismatic and they both received a warm and welcome reception wherever they went. After seeing them in action I could see why—they appeared almost like a famous comedy duo with an infectivity similar to that of the disease they were trying to educate people about.

For Michael at least, 'wrong information' was the biggest threat to him and the team achieving their target of eliminating malaria. While Danny and Renya articulated many times that people knew a lot about malaria (i.e., within a biomedical framework), at other times, they too expressed similar views that 'ignorance' or dissonant 'cultural beliefs' were issues that needed to be overcome through education. However, for Michael, education was about more than just a means to deal with infection. As he articulated, IECs were also a way to more broadly enable people to achieve what he described as 'civilisation':

The programme [from PSFI/KLM] stratifies *sitios* as civilised or not. [They are categorized as civilised] if there is a leader, a Chieftain who I can coordinate with—because some of them cannot understand how to talk Tagalog because their language is still native so it is difficult to teach those ones. Also [they are categorized as civilised] if the young people are no longer going up [pointing far off into the distance]—like they don't still have nomadic behaviour, going to the fields to do *kaingin* and instead they are in school. Also, if there is no longer the problem of going to the 'quack' doctors because they go to the RHU instead as well as other backward practices like if they are no longer getting married so young. Together, we work to uplift the IPs and empower them to change their ways to progress in all these kinds of ways through the IECs'

As a result, malaria was co-opted into Michael's strategic attempt to 'educate', 'uplift', 'civilise' and ultimately 'empower' Pälawan communities. For him, education as a means to ensure 'compliance' to science and technology went hand in hand with efforts to ensure 'compliance' to what he saw as a more 'progressive' way of life for the Pälawan. As discussed in more detail in Chap. 4, this chimed with transnational neoliberal views of economic and social development in which changes to livelihood practices, incorporation into cash economies and the uptake of education and health services were equated with growth and good governance among local government leaders in Bataraza. It is precisely this kind of 'progress' *on behalf* of Pälawan people that global medical citizens such as Danny, Renya and Michael also 'brokered' through framing and enacting malaria in the way they did.

However, as above, despite the relative consistency in the way malaria was framed as a knowable disease that could be educated about, there were also some inconsistencies that health leaders distributed out into the realm of 'individual culture', in order to avoid a clash. For example, Danny told me how he had regularly seen *balyan* (healers) using plants to successfully treat malaria in local communities, some of which he used himself. He strongly believed that these practitioners possessed effective knowledge and skills outside the realms of biomedical knowledge and practice that he and other health leaders could learn from. This was evident when I told him about meeting a particularly renowned *balyan* and he responded:

> Oh yes, I know him very well and he is a very effective *balyan*. He has a special relationship with the spirits and when I was in his house, many times, I saw him command the snakes around him showing his great power. He taught me about many kinds of plants to treat malaria and you know, when I lived up there for many months myself and it was too far to go to the RHU, I used to visit medicine men like him when I got sick and they cured my fever. Oh yes, they are very effective and have much they can teach us. They have knowledge about plants from the spirits that we do not

know about. In fact, many times people from the abroad have come here and I have taken them up to meet people because they want to try to test the plants to see if they are effective in trials to use all over the world. I have no doubt that they possess a very powerful kind of knowledge and it has saved many lives especially in the remote areas.

Despite this clear respect for 'alternative' knowledge and practices, no room was created in IECs to incorporate such expertise. Instead, Indigenous knowledge and practice was distributed into the domain of 'culture' as health leaders pushed forward with trying to achieve 'progress' by educating people about how to overcome malaria through recourse to biomedical information and practices alone.

Conclusion

As health leaders such as Danny, Renya and Michael pushed forward with their practices orientated towards different kinds of 'progress', these actors un(consciously) incorporated or distributed the malaria that was of less concern to Pälawan people, the more urgent health issues that consequently remained 'out of focus', and the knowledge and practices that Pälawan people possessed that enabled them to live healthier lives. These sentiments were expressed by many Pälawan people such as Elma, an elementary school teacher who told me:

> We will never be rid of malaria here, the mosquitoes will always be here no matter what the RHU gives us or tells us to do, they are part of this place and part of our lives. It is not our main concern anyway. What we are really concerned with are the sicknesses from the ancestors and the spirits that live in the land. These are more important. But we know how to deal with those ourselves—this is not something that the doctors in the clinic know about.

It is to the land and the sicknesses that are entangled within it that I turn to in the next chapter.

References

Adarlo, G. M. (2017). (Re)framing citizenship education in the Philippines: A twenty-first century imperative. *The Good Society, 25*(2–3), 256–288.

Anderson, W. (2007). Science in the Philippines. *Philippine Studies, 55*(3), 287–318.

Avanceña, A. L. V., Tejano, K. P. S., & Hutton, D. W. (2019). Cost-effectiveness analysis of a physician deployment program to improve access to healthcare in rural and underserved areas in the Philippines. *BMJ Open, 9*(12), e033455–e033455.

Biehl, J. o. G. (2004). The activist state: Global pharmaceuticals, AIDS, and citizenship in Brazil. *Social Text, 22*(3), 105–132.

Blaser, M. (2018). Doing and undoing Caribou/Atiku: Diffractive and divergent multiplicities and their cosmopolitical orientations. *Tapuya: Latin American Science, Technology and Society, 1*(1), 47–64.

Bossert, T., Beauvais, J., & Bowser, D. (2000). *Technical Report 1. Decentralization of health systems: Preliminary review of four country case studies.*

Bourdieu, P. (1977). *Outline of a theory of practice.* Cambridge University Press.

Brown, P. J. (1997). Culture and the global resurgence of malaria. In P. J. Brown & M. C. Inhorn (Eds.), *An anthropology of infectious disease: International health perspective.* Routledge.

Brown, P. J., & Inhorn, M. C. (1997). *An anthropology of infectious disease: International health perspectives.* Routledge.

Chandler, C., Beisel, U., Hausmann-Muela, S., Muela, J. R., & Umlauf, R. (2014). *Re-imagining malaria: Brief outputs of a workshop.* London School of Hygiene and Tropical Medicine.

DOH. (2011). *Malaria medium term development plan 2011–2016.* .

Ejercito, A., Hess, A. D., & Willard, A. (1954). The six-year Philippine-American malaria control program. *American Journal of Tropical Medicine and Hygiene, 3*, 971–980.

Espino, F., Beltran, M., & Carisma, B. (2004). Malaria control through municipalities in the Philippines: Struggling with the mandate of decentralized health programme management. *International Journal of Health Planning and Management, 19*, S155–S166.

Fassin, D. (2009). Another politics of life is possible. *Theory, Culture & Society, 26*(5), 44–60.

Iskander, D. (2015). Re-imaging malaria in the Philippines: How photovoice can help to re-imagine malaria. *Malaria Journal, 14*(1), 257.

Kelly, A. H., & Beisel, U. (2011). Neglected malarias: The frontlines and back alleys of global health. *BioSocieties, 6*(1), 71–87.

Liu, J. X., Newby, G., Brackery, A., Smith Gueye, C., Candari, C. J., Escubil, L. R., … Baquilod, M. (2013). Determinants of malaria program expenditures during elimination: Case study evidence from select provinces in the Philippines. *PLoS ONE, 8*(9).

Ministry of Health Philippines, World Health Organization, & University of California, S. F. (2014). *Eliminating malaria case-study 6: Progress towards subnational elimination in the Philippines.* .

Mol, A. (2002). *The body multiple: Ontology in medical practice.* Duke University Press.

Nading, A. M. (2013). "Love isn't there in your stomach": A moral economy of medical citizenship among Nicaraguan community health workers medical citizenship among community health workers. *Medical Anthropology Quarterly, 27*(1), 84–102.

Nguyen, V.-K. (2010). *The republic of therapy: Triage and sovereignty in West Africa's time of AIDS / Vinh-Kim Nguyen.* Duke University Press.

Packard, R. M. (1997). Malaria dreams: Postwar visions of health and development in the Third World. *Medical Anthropology, 17*(3), 279–296.

Parker, M., & Allen, T. (2014). De-politicizing parasites: Reflections on attempts to control the control of neglected tropical diseases. *Medical Anthropology: Cross-Cultural Studies in Health and Illness, 33*(3), 223–239.

Paterno, R. P. P. (2013). The future of universal health coverage: A Philippine perspective. *Global Health Governance, 6*(3).

Petryna, A. (2013). *Life exposed: Biological citizens after chernobyl* (Rev. ed.). Princeton University Press.

Romualdez Jr, A. G., dela Rosa, J. F. E., Flavier, J. D. A., Quimbo, S. L. A., Hartigan-Go, K. Y., Lagrada, L. P., & David, L. C. (2011). *The Philippines health systems review.*

Rose, N. (2007). *Politics of life itself: Biomedicine, power, and subjectivity in the twenty-first century / Nikolas Rose.* Princeton University Press.

Rose, N., & Novas, C. (2005). Biological citizenship. In A. Ong & S. J. Collier (Eds.), *Global assemblages technology, politics, and ethics as anthropological problems.* Blackwell Publishing.

Russell, P. F. (1936). Epidemiology of malaria in the Philippines. *American Journal of Public Health and the Nation's Health, 26*(1), 1–7.

Strathern, M. (1991). *Partial connections.* Rowman & Littlefield Publishers.

UCSF. (2012). *Policy brief – Funding malaria control in the Philippines: A proposal for an innovative financing mechanism.*

WHO/DOH. (2012). *Health service delivery profile – Philippines.*

Wolf, E. R. (1956). Aspects of group relations in a complex society: Mexico. *American Anthropologist, 58*(6), 1065–1078.

4

Practices of Development

Introduction

It is mid-September 2012, rainy season, and the roads are wet. Uncle Aldo
arrives with his tricycle at around 5pm and we make the 35km journey to
a guest house lobby in Rio Tuba where I am due to meet Mr Ramos, a
senior figure in the National Commission on Indigenous Peoples (NCIP).
The Puerto Princesa Road to Rio Tuba is one continuous stretch of tarmac
that hugs the full extent of the eastern edge of the island. As a minibus
driver told me on our six-hour journey south from the capital Puerto
Princesa to Bataraza, 'a lot of money has gone into this road from the government and even from foreigners. It's not for us though, going north from
Puerto, it's for the tourists and going south, it's for the mining companies—that's the story of Palawan, everything these days is for tourism and
mining.' As Aldo and I travel along the southern stretch, getting further
from Marangas and closer to Rio Tuba, the lush green of the paddy and
swidden that typically flank the road disappear, replaced by a deep red terrain with only small pockets of vegetation (and golf courses) in the distance. It is a stark contrast to the landscape that I have become used to and
impossible to miss the presence of the mining industry that is behind this
change. Fields and forest give way to vast stretches of dark exposed natural
earth and rock. The road is heaving with bulldozers, tractors and trucks

© The Author(s), under exclusive license to Springer Nature Singapore Pte Ltd. 2021   99
D. Iskander, *The Power of Parasites*, https://doi.org/10.1007/978-981-16-6764-0_4

going in and out of the Rio Tuba Nickel Mining Corporation (RTNMC). I cover my mouth with my shawl to try and prevent breathing in the air that is thick with dust and pollution. I arrive at the RTNMC Guest Lodge and send a text to Ramos; 'Hi, I am here in the lobby.' An immediate reply comes, 'Ok, just wait'. I sit in the low-lit waiting room surrounded by artificial flowers and pictures of well-known sites across Palawan with tourism slogans superimposed on in bright, friendly font; 'It's more fun in the Philippines' and '#1 for fun—Philippines'. No one comes in or out of the guest house and the receptionist idly looks at his phone for most of the time I am there. Another 25 minutes pass. I send another text 'Hi, is everything ok? We were due to meet at 6pm?' A message immediately flashes up on my screen 'Just wait.' So, I wait. Half an hour later, with Aldo still standing outside in the rain, refusing to come inside so he can continue chain smoking cigarettes, a short stocky man appears in suit trousers, a striped collared t-shirt and jacket, carrying a leather briefcase. 'Hello Dalia, I am Mr Ramos' he says in English. 'Why have you come here?' I explain my situation, that I am a research student from the UK, here to understand more about malaria among the Indigenous Pälawan. I tell him that since my initial visit to Bataraza in April that year, I had been trying to gain approvals in the Philippines to conduct my research but have been hitting obstacle after obstacle. The Institutional Review board (IRB) in the Research Institute of Tropical Medicine (RITM) were reviewing my ethics application. They advised me to contact both the Protected Area Management Board (PAMB) of the Mount Mantalingahan Protected Landscape (MMPL) and the NCIP to clarify if I needed a research permits from them as I am working in a protected conservation area and with Indigenous People. I explained to Ramos that I had already been in touch the PAMB and in accordance with their procedures, obtained Free, Prior, Informed Consent (FPIC) from the communities I planned to work in in Bataraza. I had met with community *panglimas* (leaders) and Indigenous councils from Pälawan villages and held community-wide meetings to explain my research to people and to gain their consent, as a collective, to work in their areas. I had also obtained Municipal and *barangay* resolutions from the local government. This had entailed meeting with the Mayor to secure his approval as well as numerous meetings with his secretary, Al Rajid who had, in turn, arranged meetings for me with *barangay* Captains (elected officials). While the PAMB processed my application, they told me I should ensure there wasn't anything else I needed from the NCIP. I explained that personnel in the provincial NCIP office in Puerto Princesa had given me conflicting and incomplete advice about whether or not I needed an NCIP research permit and how to go about it. They seemed united in their insistence that I had to pay uncapped stipends and expenses to fund NCIP staff travelling to the villages I wished to work in order to 'validate' the FPIC process for themselves. I told Ramos that I had come to him, as a senior figure, for clarification of the processes. Ramos sat very still as I talked and said nothing. He rested both his elbows on the arms of the chair and clasped his hands in front of his face. When I finished talking, he sighed heavily and, in a tone, that I assume was intended to intimidate me said, 'Well Dalia, the first thing you need to know is that you are here illegally. You cannot conduct research on ancestral lands or with IPs (Indigenous Peoples) without our approval. I should report you to the police and arrange for you to be thrown out of the country and sent back home. In fact, you cannot set foot on ancestral lands without our approval. You have no authority to go to these places and no authority whatsoever to hold meetings with leaders. Only we can do that. In any case, many of these *panglimas* you have met with are probably not yet validated by us so they have no real authority either. If you want to work with IPs on their land then staff from the regional office in Puerto will go there on your behalf and hold meetings with communities. You need to pay for at least three staff to go to each *barangay* you want to work in—all of their transport, hotel bills, food and a daily stipend of 800 pesos needs to be met by you. You will pay for everything they need—even if they need a ball point pen to write with, you must buy it. Filipinos are honest people; my staff will only charge you for what they use. The IPs too, they live day-to-day for food so if you want them to come to a meeting, you must provide them with their food for the day. I cannot give you any idea of how much it will cost or how long it will take. NCIP staff will validate the process of consent and send a report back to me. If I approve the research, I will draw up a contract for you to sign.' He went on, 'As well, every one of your articles or reports and thesis—anything you write has to be sent to me to validate. You cannot release any of this information to your university or publish anything until I have checked what you have written. In any case, it's dangerous for you to be here alone—a single woman like this—don't you know you can be kidnapped? People have been kidnapped here, especially if they are involved with land. You say you are here to work on malaria so why get involved with IPs and their ancestral land at all? Stick to the hospitals and clinics. The doctors and nurses there can tell you all you need to know about malaria and the IPs and you don't need any approvals to talk to them directly.' Months of frustration came to a head in this meeting. The reputation of the NCIP was one of large-scale incompetence and corruption. I had been told of many instances where the NCIP circumvented or exploited the FPIC process designed to protect IPs in return for financial benefits from pharmaceutical, mining or logging companies. I was told that ancestral land had been seized for resource extraction and clinical trials authorized to be *conducted* on people using unlicensed drugs without their consent using a mixture of bribery and deception. People I trusted had all told me the same thing—there is no clarity or consistency in processes—other than me likely having to hand over a lot of my money. The anger and upset was clear on my face. 'How do you feel now you have heard what I have to say?' Ramos asked, in the same stern but now slightly smug tone of voice. 'That this process is going to be difficult. Everyone I speak to from the PAMB or NCIP tells me something different. I am a student. I don't have a large budget to pay for all these expenses all over again. I followed the guidelines from the PAMB already to get FPIC.' I said, tears beginning to roll down my face. Ramos broke out in a sudden laugh. He relaxed his arms, leant forward and in a jovial tone said 'Oh dear, I am sorry if I have upset you. Do you have Filipino blood by any chance? I think you might because you are very sensitive like a Filipino. Don't cry. Sometimes my tone is harsh. We are here to protect the Indigenous People and their ways. I will help you, don't worry. Just text me in a few weeks to arrange everything.' And with that Ramos stood up and suddenly left. Astounded, I went outside to find Aldo and apologised for taking so long. He just laughed in his usual casual way, '*Walang problema!*' On the drive home, a text flashed up on my phone from Ramos 'Don't, worry Dalia. It will be my pleasure to serve you.' I never did get to the bottom of the process to gain a research permit from the NCIP. From then on, my colleagues in RITM communicated with them on my behalf and, in the end, confirmed I did not need to obtain any more approvals to the ones I already had. In May 2013, after a period of being at home in the UK for a few weeks, I went to the municipal office to see Al Rajid. I wanted to give him copies of my letters from the ethics committee and PAMB, the latter of which had taken over seven months to arrive. His desk was empty and I asked a colleague if he was in today. 'Oh, you haven't heard?' She asked in a surprised tone 'Al Rajid is dead'. I left in shock and asked a friend outside what had happened. 'He was killed in a shootout—shot right through the face. The bullets went into one side and came out the other. His body was shaking so much from the force of the bullets that even his baseball cap flew off his face as he was shot.' 'My gosh!' I replied, completely taken aback, 'What happened exactly?' 'Ah!' he whispered, 'The newspaper reported that Al Rajid supported Abdujarik, the main opponent of the Mayor and his wife in the election. Media[1] are saying that some supporters of the Mayor shot him in a gun battle. Another man and a 16-year-old girl were also killed. But of course, the Mayor is not directly connected. Here, everything is political but don't worry, you don't have to get involved in all that—just focus on malaria. There is no politics in that' 'If only.' I retorted 'It isn't that simple'.

In Bataraza land was a contentious issue. As the vignette above illustrates, Bataraza's Pälawan citizens that I met lived within what was demarcated as the Mount Mantalingahan Protected Landscape (MMPL). As such, the area came under the purview of a range of official actors who were invested in what they described as 'preserving' the land as well as 'protecting' the ways of life of the people who lived within it. This was in line with more recent conservation agendas that promoted ideas of participatory, community-based sustainable development (Novellino & Dressler, 2009) and the objectives of the Indigenous People's Rights Act (IPRA) of 1997 which granted IPs in the Philippines the right to self-determination over their ancestral domains. Following the fall of Ferdinand Marcos' authoritarian regime in 1986 and the transition to Corazon Aquino's Government, decentralisation and devolution meant that in the contemporary context, agencies, administrators and practitioners operated on a local level to enact preservation and protection agendas on the ground. Here, I show how the practices of local government staff within the MMPL aligned with these conservation and rights agendas as they worked towards achieving 'sustainable development'. These actors thus advocated the community-led uptake of market-orientated alternative livelihoods and sedentary farming practices in order to achieve two interrelated aims: environmental conservation and economic development. However, while staff articulated their desire to preserve and promote Indigenous ways of life, their efforts were regarded by many

---

[1] See The Philippine Star (2013).

Pälawan people as ranging from ineffectual to corrupt and as running counter to their own desires.

It is against this backdrop of global, national and regional rhetoric and practices of conservation and rights that other, locally based government officials in Bataraza operated in ways that aligned with similar agendas but implicated malaria more explicitly along the way. As a result, certain articulations of the disease were pushed forward in the name of 'development' while others were silenced. Despite the fact that much of the island had been subject to sustained, though minor, migration since the turn of the century, in the mid-twentieth century Palawan remained relatively sparsely populated due the ongoing conflicts in the south between the Tausug *datus* and the American administrators (Smith, 2020), its function as a leper and penal colony and, crucially, its endemic malaria. While contemporary government officials spoke of their intention to 'preserve' and 'protect' Indigenous lands, ways of life and rights, their practices appeared more (un)consciously orientated towards achieving other 'development' goals—namely promoting the island as a business hub for the burgeoning population of Filipino migrant settlers who had been coming to the island following World War II and, more importantly, national and international corporations pursuing opportunities in agrobusiness, tourism and mining. As such they worked towards ridding Palawan of its reputation as the most malarious island in the Philippines through strategies designed to win votes, retain political office and ultimately boost economic profit. Specifically, I describe how, in the arena of local governance, actors such as the Mayor and some *Barangay* Captains and NCIP-validated 'Chieftains' of Pälawan communities framed and enacted malaria as if it were a health problem of the 'past', eliminated due to their success at pushing forth with 'development' projects such as agroforestry, tourism and mining on ancestral lands. For them, malaria remained only in specific pockets due to lingering 'beliefs' and 'behaviours' of Indigenous People whom they felt needed to be 'developed' further to tackle this in specifically medical spheres through education and health services. However, rather than incorporate or distribute interferences as the health leaders described in Chap. 3 did, local government leaders actively refuted, denied and essentially displaced 'alternative' versions of malaria outright when they deviated from this view. In particular, versions of an emerging and enduring malaria that both health leaders and Indigenous People attributed directly to the negative and destructive environmental, social, political and economic consequences of economic activity were silenced. As such, within the field of local governance, as local officials (un)consciously worked towards gaining and retaining governmental power, the supposed eradication of malaria was lauded as a story of success of the past, demarcated into the arena of health and dismissed as an outcome of 'sustainable development'.

Sustainably Developing the Last Ecological Frontier

Governmental land management on Palawan has a long history. According to the Forest Management Bureau of the Department of Environment and Natural Resources (DENR), Palawan is the most forested province in the Philippines with approximately 690,000 hectares of woodland found in its 1,489,626 hectares total land mass.[2] The island is home to over 1600 species of flora and fauna, with numerous animals and botanical species listed in the *International Union for Conservation of Nature's* 'Red List of Threatened Species' (Sandalo & Baltazar, 1997). Dubbed the Philippines' 'last ecological frontier', the island was declared a UNESCO Man and Biosphere Reserve in 1991 and legislation passed soon after brought in a wave of changes aimed at legal environmental protection that has increasingly put the management of land in Palawan in the hands and under the scrutiny of local government (ibid.). However, along with this control has come the increased alienation of Indigenous Peoples, such as the Pälawan, from the land that their *kagurangurangan* (ancestors) occupied, largely due to the denigration of their swidden practices (*kaingin* in Tagalog and *uma* in Palawano)—a shifting and rotational cycle of slash-and-burn agriculture. As described in Chap. 2, the Spanish had already designated all non-privately titled land as 'public domain',

---

[2] Eder and Fernandez (1996) report that 90% of Palawan's land was forested at the beginning of the twentieth century, but by 2017, this had fallen to just over 40% according to figures from the Forest Management Bureau, Department of Environment and Natural Resources (DENR) (2017).

putting it under the jurisdiction of the Crown, but in reality, implementation was weak in the frontier uplands of Muslim-controlled areas such as Bataraza. However, the Americans were more successful at establishing bureaucratic infrastructure across Palawan (Smith, 2020). Land zoning began as early as 1899 (Linn, 2000) and The Kaingin Law of 1901 declared *kaingin* a severe threat to timber yields (Dressler, 2009; Scott, 1979). *Kaingineros*, as they were referred to, were considered 'squatters' and were forcibly evicted from their homes across the island or imprisoned. Following independence in 1946, and a subsequent Revised Kaingin Law in 1963, many IPs were relocated under a mandatory scheme. Condemnation of IPs and their livelihood practices continued during the Marcos Regime, now under a new paradigm of 'social forestry' under which IPs were subject to 'management and resettlement' as opposed to more punitive measures such as incarceration (Pulhin & Pulhin, 2003; Smith & Dressler, 2017). With the establishment of the Philippine Constitution of 1987, land under 18% elevation was zoned as 'alienable and disposable' and made available for the acquisition of private land titles. From the mid-twentieth century, the government offered homesteads on the 'fringes' of the archipelago in places such as Palawan to Filipinos from other parts of the country. Many migrant 'lowlanders', namely from the Visayas and Luzon took advantage, turning the land initially to swidden then permanent wet rice cultivation and later commercial agricultural use (Smith, 2020). Indigenous 'uplanders', on the other hand, were deprived of the same access to and benefits of higher elevation areas where they had conventionally lived and carried out their own forms of farming, pushed instead further into upland areas. For the Pälawan, *kaingin* and their ancestral lands are not only necessarily for nutrition, but also integral to their religious culture, livelihoods and lifeways (Dressler, 2005; Eder, 1987; Macdonald, 2007; Smith, 2018, 2020). Nevertheless, along with widespread logging that began in the Spanish period, *kaingin* was considered by many to be the primary cause of large-scale forest destruction as well as general environmental degradation (Novellino, 2000b; Suarez & Sajise, 2010). As such, governments have continued to unleash anti-swidden discourse as disciplinary, normalising practices in order to drive the adoption of permanent agriculture in the lowlands of Palawan (Dressler, 2014).

What essentially began as colonial state efforts to control land for economic productivity became intertwined, in the post-Marcos regime, with attempts to protect land for conservation purposes. In 1992, the National Integrated Protected Areas System (NIPAS), funded by the European Union (EU), had the joint aim of promoting socio-economic development as well as biodiversity conservation. Alongside it, a Strategic Environment Plan (SEP) for Palawan was adopted and the EU-funded Palawan Council for Sustainable Development (PCSD) established to oversee its implementation. With minimal state funding, the PCSD operated at arm's length from central agencies (Dressler, 2019). Under the new legal framework of the SEP, the Environmentally Critical Areas Network (ECAN) divided Palawan into zones based on elevation criteria, specifically: Terrestrial, Coastal/Marine and Tribal/Ancestral. Within each, core zones, buffer zones and multiple/manipulative use areas demarcated the land further and placed it under different levels of state purview in terms of controlled development.[3] This ranged from maximum protection, with human disruption prohibited in highest elevation core zones; medium protection, with restrictive, regulated human use allowed in buffer zones; and limited protection, with modified use and development (i.e., timber extraction, grazing, agriculture and infrastructure development) allowed in multiple/manipulative zones (Novellino, 2000a). As Dressler (2019) articulated, although difficult to enforce, this zoning system reflected a 'biopolitical "operating space" for rendering upland peoples and landscapes legible and manageable' (ibid., p. 126) by state authorities. Although ancestral lands were defined as those which have been traditionally occupied by minority groups (determined in theory by consultation with communities as discussed below), these areas were still subject to the same system of zoning and therefore control regarding their use and the subsistence methods allowed on them. Curiously, while consideration was theoretically taken to preserve Indigenous culture, no

---

[3] As Novellino (2000a) explains, core zones are defined as areas of maximum protection and consist basically of steep slopes, first growth forests, areas above 1000 meters elevation, mountain peaks and habitats of endemic and rare species. Buffer zones are the most complex but are designed to serve a multiplicity of purposes: Restricted Use Areas, Controlled Use Areas and Traditional Use Areas. Multiple/Manipulative Use Zone areas are where the landscape has been modified for different forms of land-use such as extensive timber extraction, grazing and pastures, agriculture and infrastructure development.

specific mention was made of how one of its hallmark practices—*kaingin*—could be continued, suggesting only imported methods such as terracing, hillside farming and the adoption of sedentary agroforestry practices were permitted in buffer and multiple/manipulative use zones regardless of their ancestral title (Novellino, 2000a; Smith & Dressler, 2017). Therefore, as much recent scholarship has pointed out (Dressler, 2006, 2014; Dressler et al., 2020; Dressler & Pulhin, 2010; Matsumoto-Takahashi et al., 2018; Novellino, 2000a; Novellino & Dressler, 2009; Smith, 2018, 2020; Theriault, 2017), Indigenous ways of life have continued to be jeopardised in contemporary land management. This colonial hangover has continued despite a shift in post-Marcos rhetoric towards democratisation and 'people-orientated' conservation (Novellino, 2000a). The Local Government Code of 1991 devolved authority in governance to Local Government Units (LGUs) and encouraged the active involvement of Non-Governmental Organisations (NGOs) and Civil Society Organisations (CSOs) in matters relating to conservation and land tenure in particular through community-based and participatory methods (Novellino & Dressler, 2009; Pulhin & Dressler, 2009). However, Dressler (2019) argued these non-state actors appropriated 'governmental legitimacy, authority and practices to discipline the Indigenous poor' (ibid., p. 123) in ways that position IPs as mere 'guardians' of biodiversity rather than owners or even rightful users of it. These 'biopolitical masters' (ibid) set the obligation of IPs to, at best, stabilise and, at worst, abandon their so-called destructive slash-and-burn practices in the name of economic efficiency and sustainable development (Dressler, 2019; Dressler & Pulhin, 2010). Rather than promote the extension of *kaingin*, a number of non-state agencies therefore work to encourage alternative livelihoods among IPs in Palawan such as basket making for tourism (Dressler, 2019) or promote diversification and intensification through value-added production that meets market demands (Dressler, 2014; Dressler & Roth, 2011). Schemes have encouraged a switch from long fallow to permanent cultivation through the planting of leguminous and fruit trees on fallow land to replenish soil quality, intercropping swidden with other crops that prevent soil erosion and/or turning swidden fields over altogether to monocrop paddy rice or cash-crops. This is at odds with anthropological scholarship stretching as far back Conklin's (1957, 1961) seminal work that showed how 'traditional' swidden methods actually incorporated ways of encouraging and restoring the productivity and biodiversity of the land (Cramb et al., 2009; Dressler, 2005; Dressler et al., 2017; Eder, 1997). Nevertheless, post-colonial discourses have continued to dominate conservation narratives and pit destructive, illegitimate and irrational Indigenous livelihood techniques against 'productive' lowland techniques for growing irrigated rice (Dressler, 2005).

Although the presence of NGOs and CSOs was less palpable in Bataraza than other areas of the island, the restriction of swidden and encouragement of alternative livelihoods and permanent cultivation was nevertheless present as, since 2009, the municipality was declared, by presidential proclamation, a Protected Area—the MMPL. Mount Mantalingahan was the highest peak within Palawan and its range covered a total area of 120,457 hectares within the territorial jurisdiction of the municipalities of Bataraza, Brooke's Point, Quezon, Rizal and Sofronio Espanola. In an attempt to preserve the dwindling forest, under the same zoning criteria set out by the SEP, human occupancy and land utilisation were restricted within the protected landscape. In core zones in Bataraza, the Pälawan were only able to gather forest products for ceremonial or medicinal purposes while in lower elevation buffer zones, where most now live; *kaingin* was only allowed in restricted areas that had already been turned over for such practices in the past. While many of the Pälawan I met engaged in permanent practices, such as working for minimal cash on migrant fields (*arawan* in Tagalog meaning wage labour) or even planting their own 'lowland' monocrop irrigated rice or agroforestry crops themselves, they still heavily relied on *kaingin* for their own subsistence, mixing the methods of growing culturally significant upland rice with other root, cereal and vegetable crops as described below. Within the MMPL, the Protected Areas Superintendent (PASu) was appointed to implement the SEP and oversee operations while a Protected Areas Management Board (PAMB) had oversight through representatives from various sectors including business, agriculture, NGOs and Indigenous People. As the PASu explained to me, their collective remit was to support 'sustainable development' through working with a range of actors in the community to encourage 'alternatives' to *kaingin* that both supposedly benefited the environment and the people economically and in terms of livelihood:

> We involve the communities and tell them not to make their *kaingin* in new places because it is one of the main ways that the virgin forest is being destroyed. Oh yes, we want to preserve their culture so they can make their *kaingin* in some places but now it is limited so they do not destroy the primary forest. We have so many livelihood projects including those run by NGOs that show them better ways to live that in the end are good for them to get food and money. So, slowly we are educating those IPs.

While the PASu articulated that these changes were 'good' for the Pälawan, the sentiment was not shared by many people I spoke to who complained of dwindling yields and unwanted changes to lifeways that they stated had been passed down for generations. As Oket, who lived in the *sitio* of Inogbong, showed me his *kaingin* field one dry September day, he explained how practices had changed in direct response to government control:

> We learnt these ways from our *kagurangurangan* (ancestors). Before, you would have to identify the area in the forest where you want to do you *kaingin*. Usually, it is about half a hectare and it is this shape [indicates the rectangular shape of his field] but it doesn't need to be flat. The first thing to do is many prayers to ask permission from *diwata* (spirits) who own trees or plants before you disturb that place. There are many stages starting in December or January when the *bulag* (dry season—December/January-March/April) has started and the winds are hot. We clear the area of plants and trees and then do *duruk* (burning) of the area by March and then after March prepare for the second *duruk*. That means all the trees left from the first *duruk* are collected and put in a pile and burned so there is nothing left. After the second *duruk*, you leave the ash to feed the soil. Before the *barat* (wet season between May-December) begins and the first rain will fall it must be done but sometimes it is difficult if the rain comes early or very late. In any case, you must try to do *tugdaq* (sewing) before the rain comes. You must pray to *Ampu at paray* (Master of the rice) and to the *kagurangurangan* to ensure that there is not too much rain or heat and the harvest is good. We make *ungsud* (offerings)—you can make a *pinadungan*

(small wooden 'seat' made from woven palm) in the middle of the *uma* (swidden field) for the *paray* (rice) seeds or just put them on a plate and leave them there the night before you are ready to plant. The next day we [usually related male kin/neighbours] use the *tugdaq* (dibble stick) to make a little hole and the women put the *paray* seeds in hole. The first step is to fill the *uma* with different varieties of *paray* in rows. Many kinds of *paray* can be planted in a half hectare. We have short-term and long-term harvest types—some come after three months but *maitoniton* (black rice) and *binato* (red rice) come later. Next you plant the *ubi* (purple yam) which needs to climb up the stems of trees. You can also plant *meis* (corn) at the same time as the *paray*. The second step is to plant *bugbubug* (cassava) in lines. Here [pointing], in the corner you will segregate the *sanglay* (sweet potatoes, also often referred to as *kamote* in Tagalog) which has a long vine. You can put the *aturay* (millet) in the boarder. You cannot plant that inside with the *paray* as it is jealous. If you put them together it will not grow or they will grow so much that the *paray* will die. Sometimes we have *kadyos* (beans) and *tales* (taro, also often referred to as *gabi* in Tagalog), whatever you like can go in the boarder and *punti* (banana) and *niyug* (coconut) trees are all around. Then, there is much weeding and caretaking to do. By September everything is finished here except some *kadyos, gabi* and *ubi* and then you leave it as *bangley* (fallow) for one or two years. But you can come back and keep claiming the *bugbubug, punti or nlyug* from the trees—that is still yours. These will keep growing for a year or even more—the *niyug* for even seven years. We keep it for a life time this way. But now, the MMPL said, 'no you cannot burn or plant any more in a new area up there after you harvest from here'. When they say 'up there', it doesn't even mean in the forbidden area where the very big trees are, the virgin forest, it's even just a little bit up there. All the *kaingin* has to be done in a certain area. So now, we do *palyud* (second *kaingin*) too—we do not burn in that area but we just clear the weeds and scatter the rice straw like a fertilizer in an area that we have used before. It's similar to *kaingin* but we have to grow different *paray* and other plants because the soil is not so good. It's hard now to make *kangin* in the old way. All people have *kaingin* and *palyud*. Even though we don't have a good yield we continue but the yield is getting less and less. That's why a few people are even trying the lowland rice or growing fruits and other things to sell. Not all people want to do that as it is changing our ways so they keep doing *kaingin* and maybe work as *arawan* for some money. They [the government] have divided the land but in some areas they still don't have a concrete plan so some are still doing *kaingin* in places illegally like in Bonobono because it isn't clear what is the plan. Here in Inogbong, they have already divided the land. They have designated a core zone where you can't do any activities there. We used to move around a lot to do our *kaingin* to get high yields but now things have changed because of the government and so we stay here only.

Although sustainable development for the PASu meant promoting alternative livelihood projects with the 'involvement' of the community, talking to people like Oket made it clear that initiatives were far from inclusive and had very little reach in some areas. For example, Smith (2018) and Smith and Dressler et al. (2017) document how one particular community-based agroforestry project in the *barangay* of Inogbong only benefited some, leading to palpable divisions when their fieldwork was conducted in 2011–2012. Initiated by the PCSD in 1995, the seven-year project named the Palawan Tropical Forest Protection Program (PTFPP) was funded by the EU. Its aim was to promote fixed forms of market-oriented agroforestry alongside alternative forms of income generation in order to stall deforestation. As an alternative to *kaingin*, the planting of high-value, perennial and 'enriching' trees and vegetables (e.g., cashew, kalamansi lime, mango, lakatan bananas and rattan) that were grown in nurseries set up around the *barangay* was promoted. In return for planting them, community members were reimbursed with cash as well as clothes, utensils, food and radios. In many ways, the project aimed to lock upland farmers into place, not so much by demarcating boundaries but by socialising them into alternative ways of life (ibid.). As Smith and Dressler et al. (2017) explain, in the spirit of community-based forest management, the project included the recruitment of willing *panglimas* and respected community members to act as 'brokers' in promoting ideas about how certain activities (e.g., swidden and the extraction of forest products/wildlife) were environmentally, economically and morally detrimental through a series of information dissemination campaigns. The authors show how many in the community were brought 'on board' with the idea that permanent trees were of high value, in need of protection and that sedentary and newer practices were indeed better than swidden. However, they point out that while the project seemed to reach and have benefits for those living in lower elevations, many inhabitants living in the more remote uplands of the *barangay* felt little positive buy-in and impact from the project. As such, the promise of 'sustainable development' was only for the few (ibid.). Similarly, Dressler (2019) describes how the NGO, Conservation International, implemented Community Conservation Agreements in areas including Bataraza, employing local farmers and community members to act as rangers, tasked with monitoring and preventing the opening of new forest for swidden. In exchange, other 'traditional' practices were promoted for income generation such as the weaving of *tingkep* lidded baskets, imbued as they were with *diwata* (spirits) and forest patterns, for tourist consumption. Through *re-making* the *tingkep* weaving custom as a means to incentivise sedentism, Dressler (2019) argues, the project simultaneously *unmade* another fundamental dimension of Pälawan life—shifting *kaingin*. Similar sentiments were held by people I spoke to concerning these two projects but I did not hear of or see any others initiated within the MMPL by either state or non-state organisations in my time in Bataraza. Overall, the reputation of the PCSD and PAMB in particular was of ineffectiveness at best and corruption at worst. As one of my friends who used to work in the municipal office, Yorick, who was familiar with PTFPP articulated, motives were questionable:

> For example, the EU came here in the Philippines to preserve the whole of Palawan especially the forested area. That was 20 years ago. They set aside millions of dollars for that and asked the Philippines to be a counterpart of 100 million pesos only. This was when the PCSD was established. They built a very nice building in Puerto Princesa and bought many luxury Land Rovers from England. I think they were 1.5 million pesos each and they bought maybe 28 of them so can you imagine that cost. The money of the EU went on those expenses and the salary of the staff. Even the driver had a monthly income of 21,000–30,000 pesos and the casual workers and directors had a very big salary. According to them, the major goal was, number one, indirect programmes and then number two, direct programmes. The indirect programme were projects like goat raising, cow fattening, communal gardening, reforestation. That means talk to the people doing illegal *kaingin* and illegal loggers and tell them to do an alternative livelihood like that instead. The direct programme was establishing check

points to check illegal loggers and all the logistics like radio handsets and an information drive about the environment and giving authority to forest rangers. But, you know, as far as my experience is concerned, the indirect and direct programme had a very small effect on the community. The goal of the programmes was defeated. We started a lot of projects but they were not sustainable. That is the reason it failed. When the EU sent consultants to evaluate the project and they saw it was a big failure they stopped the money. The money was not being used properly here and so some of it was returned. The number one reason for failure was the sincerity of the motive. If the motive was to protect the environment, the people and situation of the island then it would work but instead they are only interested in money. They don't want to help the island of Palawan and the people. They just want work for themselves and money.

When I asked Yorick how this and similar projects had been received among Pälawan communities, he gave a damning indictment:

[laughs] What a question! Well, on the radio you hear them all the time saying they help the tribal people and preserving the culture by providing alternative livelihoods. But when you go to the interior to places in Bataraza and you ask them, 'do you hear anything about the projects of the MMPL or PCSD, even the PAMB?', they say they have never even heard of them or seen people from those organisations come to them even though they living right there in the heart of the areas of their projects. How can that be? In my opinion, there is no good impact on the communities at all.

This chimed with the attitudes of many Pälawan people I spoke to. As Oket explained above, the laws and rules relating to *kaingin* practices remained ambiguous to those on the ground with little clarity on how land had been demarcated and could be used officially. Furthermore, the spirit of 'community-based' resource management had little material impact and, crucially, had not changed the view among people that restrictions were still essentially punitive, coercive and in no way aligned with maintaining their ways of life (Eder, 1997; Smith, 2018).

Uncertainty and fear were particularly exacerbated by the fact that people compared the restrictions put on their own practices to business activities on land that are sanctioned by the PCSD and PAMB. For example, one lady, Nernas, told me:

> The authorities tell us not to make *kaingin* up there in some places and not others but we have been here since time immemorial so we already know not to cut the big trees. We are scared people are watching us and we will go to prison. Now, we are forced to only make *kaingin* in the same places. They say it's ok to just grow *sanglay* (sweet potato) but now the *paray* (rice) is not enough for us. We know to leave it time to grow (fallow). But it is the same people that let the mining and logging companies here to take what they want without our agreement. They are allowed to come and this is the big cause of our problems because they take what is here and cut the big trees or places with *diwata* that we know not to cut and do they go to prison? No. They are all, you know, how to say … corrupt.

As a result, while commitments were ostensibly made by state actors within the MMPL to align development agendas with preserving the needs and wishes of the Pälawan, in reality, land zoning represented an ambiguous continuation of the threats posed to consultation, self-determination and rights over land and resources. This ran directly at odds with the tenants of the IPRA as discussed in the next section.

The Right to Self-determination

In 1997, the Philippines Congress enacted the IPRA which recognised and promoted the rights of Indigenous Cultural Communities/ Indigenous Peoples to self-determination. A fundamental principal was that it provided mechanisms for the recognition and protection of Indigenous ancestral domains and all resources therein. The IPRA built on policy shifts ushered in with the 1987 Constitution a decade earlier that left behind ideas of assimilation and integration in favour of recognition and preservation (Magno & Gatmaytan, 2013). Accordingly, in 1993, a Special Order was enacted by the Department of Environment and Natural Resources (DENR) to create a task force responsible for identifying, delineating and recognising ancestral domains and claims.

The NCIP that was established to implement the IPRA was tasked with processing claims through a newly upgraded land tenure mechanism called the Certificate of Ancestral Domain Title (CADT). This would theoretically give title holders *de facto* ownership rights over forests, Non-Timber Forest Products (NTFP) and *de jure* holdings over land (Dressler et al., 2012). However, as many Pälawan people told me, similar to my own experiences described above in trying to obtain a research permit from the NCIP, the CADT process was extremely complicated, opaque, bureaucratic, expensive and mired in reports of corruption and scandal. As a result, while a few certificates had been granted in areas that I worked in in Bataraza, many applications remained outstanding, in contention or never fully got off the ground. Crucially for the vast majority of people that I met, the CADT process was misaligned with Pälawan customary laws and practices pertaining to both land 'ownership' and 'consent'.

Central to the IPRA was the adoption of the concept of 'Free and Prior Informed Consent' (FPIC) as a means to supposedly protect Indigenous rights and interests by giving IPs the ability to sanction issues that affected them. In doing so, it theoretically challenged state monopoly of the exercise of law by recognising the validity and effectiveness of Indigenous legal systems in resolving issues such as disputes, the identification of ancestral domains, decisions regarding the exploitation of resources on ancestral lands (Magno & Gatmaytan, 2013) as well as involvement with academic researchers such as myself. The IPRA also, in theory, achieved an important counterbalance to much of the conservation rhetoric discussed above that vilified *kaingin*. It supposedly abandoned the perception that swidden farming caused the degradation of forest and gave IPs legal recognition over their land and crucially, what they did with it, including *kaingin* if they so desired (ibid.). However, theory did not seem to translate into practice. In reality, the Pälawan living in Bataraza continued to face innumerable obstacles aligning their views and wishes with 'foreign' templates for land tenure and ownership as well as in realising their right to even give or withhold FPIC in matters relating to their lives.

When speaking to staff from the NCIP, it was clear that the language and agenda of rights intermingled with that of sustainable development. Just as Mr Ramos had articulated above, another NCIP staff member told me, their aim was to 'help protect the rights of the IPs who have their own ways of doing things that need to be preserved in order that they can develop in a way they want'. However, aligning with and enacting what Pälawan people wanted seemed more of an expressed ideal by NCIP staff than an actuality. For example, when it came to the CADT process, many Pälawan articulated that the concept of 'ownership'—imbued as it is with ideas related to biodiversity and elevation—did not align with their own conceptions of land-use and occupation based on matrilocal residence, paternal inheritance, borrowing among kin and the sharing of resources among collectives. As one young Pälawan man explained to me:

> When I married, I moved to live with my wife's family in another *sitio* (village). … Her parents gave us some of their land to build our own house and do our own *kaingin*. That is land that their ancestors gave to them. In time, if I want to give this land to my relative, say my cousin, I can do so. I can say to him, 'You see that coconut plantation over there, that is yours now and you can take all the *niyug* (coconut fruits) from it, but I will still come and take the palms'. Or I might say 'You can take the *paray* (rice) but I will come and take the *punti* (bananas) for me and my wife and children'. It is no problem to borrow land from your family like that or to share what is there between us as we decide.

As such, as Novellino (2000c) describes, 'Indigenous communities do not perceive of themselves as either individual claimants or owners and do not refer to their land in terms of tenure, commodity, survey plans, sketch maps and sworn statements' (ibid., p. 62). Rather, landscapes are communally occupied and shared in ways that cross spatial and temporal boundaries as well as the margins between life and death (human and non-human). As discussed in a lot more detail in Chaps. 5 and 6, within Pälawan cosmology, land is seen by many to be imbued with unseen entities including dead ancestors, dwarves, giants and crucially *diwata* (spirits). The latter are conceived of as not just inhabiting but also 'owning' features of the landscape such as the earth, trees, rocks, plants and so on. Humans are inextricably linked to their environments as they continuously work towards peacefully co-existing with these 'masters' with whom they share their environments. It is customary, for example, for people to ask the permission from *diwata* before using the land for swidden or harvesting plants for medicinal use as Oket explained earlier. *Diwata* are appeased through regular offerings or prayer and omens to take care or beware are seriously heeded. A symbiotic and reciprocal relationship between humans and the unseen inhabitants of the land is therefore conceived of. Many people told me that the process to obtain land titles is fraught with difficulty as, in order to 'prove' they have 'owned' the land from time immemorial, claimants had to submit testimonials from elders, documents, maps and drawings of how the land was conceived of and used, as well as genealogies and political structures—a kind of evidence-base which did not fit with the customary practices described above. Consequently, there was very little faith in the NCIP and their ability to 'validate' the claims for titles. Similar to my own experience with the NCIP, many Pälawan people told me they were asked to finance stipends for personnel to authenticate their claims—personnel who they had heard also doubly claimed stipends back from the NCIP. A local Pastor who had helped some groups to process claims explained the situation he had witnessed many times:

> The NCIP is useless. It is a stagnant office. Not only that, when they arrive here, they will ask money from the *panglimas* and people and say they have no money to go back and no money for the gasoline for their motor and you know all the pitiful people here will dig into their pockets and gather all their little money that has been saving for months to buy coffee or pay school fees and give it to the NCIP officer. It is a disgrace.

These issues were exacerbated by the fact that the NCIP were in the process of reorganising social structures, instating validated 'Chieftains' to govern *barangays*. Like the pastor above, Ramil had extensive experience working with Pälawan communities and explained to me the problem of the Chieftain validation process in relation to what the Pälawan regard to be their customary systems of government:

> Before, there was a lot of conflict between the tribes but I will call this 'normal conflict' like about the boundaries of which tree someone is able to take fruit from … but right now, through the NCIP, there is a lot of what I call 'man-created conflict'. … It is because in the past there was no

'Chieftains' for them. You cannot find this position in the traditional culture of the people here. This has been created by the local NCIP office here in Palawan and people are really not happy about it. Now, because of that confusion, there are two types of leader at this time. The Chieftains are appointed through the government through the NCIP. But the *panglimas*, they are not under the government or NCIP—they are part of the inherited culture. According to the rules of the NCIP, they will identify those tribal people who have a royal bloodline then validate them, putting them in the positions as Chieftain only if they can really validate their claims to the bloodline and if they have the support of enough families. … Each Chieftain must have 40–50 families supporting them. So, if I am a *panglima* with a royal bloodline and 40–50 families under me then I am eligible to become a Chieftain but if I am a *panglima* with a bloodline and only 30 families under me then I cannot become a Chieftain by the NCIP. If you cannot validate your bloodline or you do not have enough families to support you then maybe you will become one member of the council of the Chieftain who is eventually validated. There is a chance of that because the Chieftain has to appoint a tribal council of tribal police, a secretary, a treasurer and a tribal advisor and so on so maybe he will choose you or maybe he will not. Anyway, who will the people follow? As you can see, this validation is causing conflicts between people.

One *panglima*, Nalde, whose position was disputed by the NCIP, added to this picture of complexity, as he described the historically contingent nature of the use of the term *panglima*. He explained how this was taken up by the Pälawan as recently as 1964 when Bataraza become a separate municipality to the neighbouring one of Brookes Point and was reorganised into *sitios*. As Smith (2018) explains Tausug *datus* were gradually incorporated into the new bureaucratic infrastructure of the southern municipal government increasing the social and economic dislocation of the Pälawan even further as the uplands and the people inhabiting them became spaces to be actively managed. Alongside this, as *panglima* Nalde described, NCIP-validation was another form of governance that circumvented the nature of land, inherited titles and the ways in which decisions were made:

Originally, we did not even use the term *panglima*. When the Muslims were in charge, they divided us into areas called *sitios* and told us we must have a leader for each *sitio* and to call it a *panglima*—that is a Muslim way of calling it. This was the time of the first Mayors—*datu* Sapiodin Narrazid and then Hadjes Asgali. Before them, we just had a *gungurang* which means oldest respected person in the community and we would just follow him and obey him. He was a lone leader and would teach morals and values and would have good qualities of leadership. He must know the *adat* (customary law) and be a master of *bitsara* (debating) in order to lead the people and teach them well. So, the *gungurang* is similar to the *panglima* you could say but the other positions that are now enforced by the NCIP are not used by us at all—there is no equal to that. They [council positions] come from another group, the Tagbanua, but the NCIP just told us we must have a council like them even though this is not from *our own* culture. In some places, if the NCIP has put in a Chieftain, the people may follow him but only if he is respected by them already as their *panglima*. In other places, it has created many problems. Like here, my grandfather was commanding this whole area and recognised by all the people as *panglima*. Even now, if we have too much sunshine, we will get oil from a coconut tree facing east together with black rice and take it to his grave to appease him. If there is too much rain then we take white rice. He is recognised as the *panglima* even though he has died already. When he was about to die, he leant the title to my father-in-law because at that time, he was the most respected older man because my own father was still young. When both my father-in-law and my father died, the position went to my uncle and then when he died, to me. Now there is a conflict with the NCIP over who has the official bloodline of *panglima*. It was my father—the position was just borrowed by my father-in-law but the NCIP say, 'no you cannot borrow positions'. So now, they recognise my in-law's family not my own bloodline. So, I am only *panglima* for this area up to the mango plantation, not the whole *barangay*. Even though the people chose to follow me here, the other man is the official Chieftain set by the government. When we have to make decisions about young people marrying or if there are too many sunny days, they come to me not him because they recognise me as their *panglima*. In some other areas, the Chieftains are also corrupt. They just work for the government and allow them to take the land for money, for example for mining. They are not recognised by the people at all, maybe they even work for the government or come from a different place altogether. In that case, the people will still go to their *panglima* when an issue needs resolving and we do it according to *adat*.

The tensions in communities created by the NCIP and their validation processes of both land and leadership titles were palpable and testament to the difficulties that many Pälawan faced in trying to achieve the 'self-determination' promised by the IPRA. As described below, these issues were pertinent to understanding how malaria was discursively conceived of and practically dealt with among officials from or linked to the municipal government in Bataraza. In their hands, the disease was intertwined with attempts to 'develop' the municipality and its people, ostensibly in line with the sustainability and rights agendas discussed so far.

'A thing of the past'

It was August 2012. I had been in Bataraza for a matter of days but had been told repeatedly by my contacts in the Rural Health Clinic [RHU] that before I began any research, I had to seek approval and a Municipal Resolution from the Mayor. Ramil arranges and accompanies me to a meeting in the municipal building in the centre of Marangas. We enter the Mayor's office in which he sits at his large wooden desk surrounded by five or six other men who are not introduced to me. Ramil and the Mayor have a jovial conversation in Tagalog that I deduce from subsequent conversations with Ramil relates to his application to the NCIP to be a municipal council representative for Indigenous People in Bataraza. The Mayor is a small, quietly spoken man and talks courteously and politely to me in English, welcoming me to Bataraza and asking me about my research. We speak for an hour and he is keen to tell me that President [Benigo] Aquino's health policies are his 'top priority'. He explains, 'there used to be a lot of malaria here in Palawan but in Bataraza, this is becoming a thing of the past. It is my personal mission to rid us of malaria completely especially among the Indigenous Peoples here in Bataraza.' I ask the Mayor what has been behind this success. He replies, 'I have diverted a lot of my own personal money in health since I have become Mayor. When they need them, I give the RHU my own cars and boats and places to stay to go to conduct their medical missions in the very hard to reach areas where we still have a few people with malaria … but you know, the main reason is investment. Since I have become Mayor, Bataraza has become a first-class municipality because of all the activities we are doing here this is providing work for the IPs. Some of the beliefs and behaviours of the natives are how to say, keeping malaria, but now they have many more opportunities for their livelihoods. You will see for yourself what we have here to lift people here out of their situation.' As we continue talking, the Mayor offers me 'whatever help [I] need' for [my] stay. 'I will give you a security guard to travel with you since you are a woman here on your own and you could be kidnapped'. Despite having read the news reports of foreign nationals being kidnapped by criminal and terrorist groups and the high number of killings of environmental activists elsewhere in the country, I decline his offers for security and thank him for his support in processing my Resolution to conduct my research. Before I leave, he says something to the men sitting around him in Tagalog that I do not catch. As we leave, Ramil turns to me with a laugh, 'Ah he told those men, "Don't bother her or let anybody else bother her. She is my guest here—help her in any way she needs."'

During my time in Bataraza, it became obvious that it was impossible to understand the nature of malaria in the area without understanding its contextualisation within wider political agendas and the players that enacted them. In the municipal structure, the most important figure was the Mayor who, in the devolved system of government, had supervision and control over all health programmes, projects and services (Espino et al., 2004). The *Sangguniáng Bayan* (Municipal Council) was the local legislative branch (presided over by the Vice-Mayor and constituted elected councillors including the representative for Indigenous Peoples). They were responsible for passing ordinances and resolutions for the administration of the municipality such as the ones I needed for my research. Each of the 22 *barangays*—the smallest political units—had their own legislative office—*the Sangguniang Barangay*. This was composed of one elected *Punong Barangay* (*Barangay* Captain), a group of elected *Barangay Kagawads* (*Barangay* Councillors) and the Chairman of the *Sangguniang Kabataanor* (Youth Assembly). In addition, although they held no legislative or executive power, NCIP-validated Chieftains had some sway over decision-making on behalf of the Pälawan communities they represented. Here, I describe how actors such as the Mayor and some *Barangay* Captains and NCIP-approved Chieftains framed and dealt with malaria in tandem with their efforts to 'develop' Bataraza and 'lift' the lives of its citizens.

In the Philippines, municipalities are divided into income classes according to their average annual income during the last three calendar years. On this rating, Bataraza was ranked within the wealthiest category as a 'first-class' municipality and had an annual income of at least 55 million Philippine Pesos (approximately £800,000). As the Mayor described, this rating was achieved during his time in office and was no doubt attributed to the substantial investment he presided over in the areas of infrastructure and industry. The principal sources of economic capital were fishing, agrofarming and nickel mining and processing with logging, oil drilling and eco-tourism also playing an increasingly important role. This was to the extent that many of the older migrant settlers in Bataraza felt that they were now being governed or pushed out by the influx of national and international business opportunists as intimated by the minibus driver quoted at the start of the chapter. It was agrofarming and mining that had the most significant impact in terms of malaria. In the case of farming, as described above, *kaingin* was actively dissuaded within the MMPL. Instead, alienable and disposable land in the lowlands was increasingly been turned over to cash-crop plantations, namely paddy rice, rubber, coconuts, copra (dried coconut shells) and cashew nuts. However, since the first palm oil seedlings were planted on the island in 2007 (Dressler et al., 2018), a growing amount of such land in Bataraza was being been used for palm oil production, the outputs of which were sold to Singapore, Malaysia and China (Larsen et al., 2014). As Larsen et al. (2014) have argued, palm oil cultivation and the promotion of private sector agro-business in Palawan formed 'part of the national government's objective to reduce palm oil imports and seize production shares in the international market' (ibid., p. 15) and was justified by local government officials as a productive use of the municipalities' supposedly abundant but 'vacant or idle lands' (ibid.). Production on the island was conducted by the Palawan Palm & Vegetable Oil Mills, Inc. (PPVOMI) (which was 60% Singaporean-owned and 40% Filipino) and its sister company Agumil Philippines, Inc. (AGPI) (which was 75% Filipino-owned and 25% Malaysian). Titled land owners had established contracts with PPVOMI and AGPI, either as independent self-financed land owners or through the use of two cooperatives in Bataraza (who organised manpower). While land owners and cooperative members tended to be migrant 'lowlanders', many Indigenous Pälawan were employed in *arawan* (Tagalog for wage labour) to carry out plantation work such as maintenance, harvesting or working as so-called loose fruit-ers (i.e., workers that picked over-ripe fruit that has fallen to the ground) for a minimum wage of around PHP 210 per day (ibid.). As of 2014, production areas were estimated to be at least 4500 hectares with future expansion planned at more than 10,000 hectares in southern Palawan (Montefrio, 2017). As well as agroindustry, more than half of Bataraza's residents were employed by the Rio Tuba Nickel Mining Corporation (RTNMC) and mineral processing plant Coral Bay Nickel Corporation (CBNC), Philippine and Japanese corporations who were the major driv-ers of economic development in Bataraza contributing billions to the economy each year. As the Mayor alludes to, these 'alternative livelihood' options were actively encouraged as a means to reduce malaria among the Pälawan by diminishing *kaingin* and the associated 'beliefs and behav-iours' that supposedly sustained transmission.

As well as encouraging agroforestry and mining, one way that the Mayor planned to boost Bataraza's economic profile even further was to turn it into the 'tourist capital of the South' as he called it to attract 'more foreigners like [myself]' and create yet more alternative livelihood oppor-tunities. In Southern Palawan, tourism was not as thriving an industry compared to the north of the island due to its less pristine coastline, lack of infrastructure, reputation as a seat of Islamist separatism and, of course, its malaria incidence. However, Bataraza was becoming a more popular site for (mainly domestic) tourists due to the Kapangyan and Lalutan Falls and Gangub Cave located there. The neighbouring municipality of Brooke's Point was trying to establish its reputation as an eco-tourist hub in Southern Palawan—something that officials in Bataraza were also keen to emulate in order to exploit the potential from the 1.4 million foreign tourists and 4 million domestic tourists that descended on Palawan island each year. The construction of an airport was planned in the near future in Brooke's Point and the Mayor talked of his ambition to build hotels, roads and a number of tourist attractions to cater for the visitors that he hoped would also flock to Bataraza. However, he was particularly worried that the reputation of southern Palawan, as the 'malaria capital' (Ramos, 2013) of the Philippines presented an obstacle to his intentions. As he went on:

> People do not want to come to a place if there is malaria but I am glad to say we are so close to completely eliminating malaria from Bataraza. That will of course help the IPs as well. With these initiatives, we can give a final push to help the communities that still have it. There is malaria in some of those very remote places because the IPs there still move around a lot into the deep forest. The way they do their farming means they do not stay in one place all year round. Providing alternative livelihoods will help with that. Where malaria remains, the RHU are doing a lot to tackle that with their missions. They are educating them and giving out things like free nets and drugs.

Consequently, the Mayor's motivations for investing in malaria control and elimination appeared deeply intertwined with his economic ambitions for the area. However, in lauding the successes of controlling malaria for and through economic development, actors such as the Mayor simultaneously refuted and even denied claims made by health staff and Pälawan communities that these activities were themselves the direct source of dislocation, hardship and disease transmission. For example, in the case of palm oil, as Larsen et al. (2014) explain, many cooperatives received loans from the Land Bank of the Philippines under the so-called Development Advocacy Program, in order to fund their contractual obligations. Although land titles were theoretically reviewed and confirmed by the bank, prior to lending, many Indigenous People alleged the process was ineffectual or corrupt and that their ancestral lands were wrongly seized and appropriated in the process, depriving them of their rightful determination. In my own work, health staff and Pälawan people reported both land grabbing, ill-health and a rise in malaria cases in particular due to land-use changes, especially mining. Unsurprisingly, this was at odds with narratives from company staff and representatives. As described above, the corporations in Bataraza conducted a range of Corporate Social Responsibility (CSR) activities through the non-stock, non-profit

Rio Tuba Nickel Foundation Incorporation (RTNFI). This was in line with government regulation that, since the 1995 Mining Act was passed, stipulated 1% of direct mining and milling costs should be allocated to Social Development and Management Programmes. The RTNFI set aside a budget of PHP 90 million to be spent over five years, and oversaw the building of a 30-bed capacity hospital to provide free healthcare to employees of the company and residents of the 11 *barangays* closest to the mines, what were referred to as 'Impact Areas'. Free education was delivered to children in these areas through the Leonides S. Virata Memorial private Catholic school as well as financial support given to teachers to work with out-of-school pupils within the Alternative Learning System. Permanent houses were built in cooperation with the NGO, Gawad Kalinga Community Development Foundation, Inc. (GK) that began in 1999 through the Couples for Christ Catholic lay ecclesiastical movement whose goal was to renew and strengthen Christian values. On an initial scoping visit to Bataraza in April 2013, I visited the Foundation in Rio Tuba to see the 'GK villages' as they were referred to for myself (Gawad Kalinga meaning 'to give or award care'). On a tour of one of these areas, there was certainly a lot to look at. Colourful brick houses circled a central sports field where children played basketball. A water pump provided fresh water for drinking and cleaning and a generator was installed for electricity. All the houses had metal roofs which likely reduced the number of mosquitoes able to get into living spaces and survive the hot temperatures indoors, and windows were screened with netting while new-looking mosquito nets hung over beds. I was told that RTNFI had gained FPIC from the Chieftain and community who had been living in the area to buy their ancestral land. The company had cleared the land of trees and vegetation, built access roads and a number of support buildings before blasting the areas with dynamite to open up quarries for limestone used in nickel processing. Although the Chieftain had used money from this sale to buy land close by upon which to relocate himself and his immediate family, others had 'chosen' to remain in the area and, after their houses were destroyed, became beneficiaries of the GK houses we were viewing. It was obvious the Foundation representative that I was with did not want me to speak with residents directly but was keen to tell me herself how happy they were to be in receipt of such housing, services such as water and electricity, education and—crucially—healthcare. Despite the claims I had heard that land had been appropriated by the Foundation under duress, she was adamant that mining and associated CSR activities had improved the health and well-being of the residents in the GK village, especially in relation to malaria. Consequently, although there was tacit recognition of the negative effects of mining through the very existence of CSR activities, senior representatives of the Foundation in particular underplayed or denied these, instead highlighting their success in 'empowering' communities to live 'healthy and sustainable' lives by integrating them into an 'urbanised' world that they felt would be especially important once the mines closed down and the corporations had left. In a meeting with a senior member of the Foundation, I was told in no uncertain terms that I was not welcome to conduct my research with IP communities who were beneficiaries of the CSR projects if my objective was to 'investigate people's lies about the supposed negative health effects of mining companies in order to mobilize them to raise up their voices in protest'. The irony that the very people he claimed to be empowering were the same ones he was simultaneously silencing seemed to be lost on him (or at least conveniently pushed to one side).

Some of the *Barangay* Captains of the 11 *barangays* in Impact Areas similarly underplayed or even actively denied the potential adverse health effects of mining in discussions I had with them. On the whole, they were in agreement that CSR activities were of real benefit to their constituents. As one Captain put it:

> The company does a lot for the people here. As well as jobs and livelihoods, the Foundation gives them free health care if you work for them and they have many nice programmes for better housing and giving bed nets for example. All of this has helped us to develop this place and rid it of malaria. It is overall very good for people's health. It is not true that mining has created more malaria here. In fact, it is the opposite—through all these programmes.

However, according to health workers and community members, it was not in the interests of Captains in Impact Areas to publicly denounce the actions of Corporations lest they lose their financial support and investment. Some people that I spoke to in the communities directly affected were also of the opinion that their *Barangay* Captains had received personal bribes from mining companies explaining that this was the 'real' reason why they sanctioned the destruction of ancestral lands under their jurisdiction. For these actors, lauding the success of malaria control and elimination as a direct result of economic development and CSR activities was therefore arguably a strategy for promoting their own public and potentially private economic interests as well as a mechanism for holding onto governmental power.

Similar motivations appeared to be behind why some NCIP-validated Chieftains also ostensibly supported mining activities on ancestral domains. While some had a more ambivalent attitude towards the changes, a couple were keen to tell me that they had agreed to extraction on their land because it brought many benefits to their communities, helping to 'develop', 'improve' or 'modernise' them as one put it:

> Now we can feed our children and send them to school thanks to those companies. Before, we didn't have ways to earn money but now we do. They gave us nice houses to live and even radios. We can go to the hospital when we get sick. Sure, it has changed our ways of life but for many of us, we have modernised and have been shown better ways to live.

However, similar to *Barangay* Captains, some of the Chieftains who had been validated by the NCIP were also the subject of scandal, with rumours circulating that they too had personally profited from selling land, both in terms of gaining their NCIP endorsement and in terms of receiving large financial rewards in return. Worse still, some were said to be decoys, delegitimate leaders or outsiders from the community altogether, brought in to work in direct cahoots with the NCIP to displace rightful leaders who opposed mining. This echoed stories in the media from other areas in Palawan that claimed 'fake leaders' had been sent to Manila by mining companies and the NCIP to support extractive activities on the island (Balana, 2011). As one 'lowlander' friend told me:

It is terrible that mining is happening in the ancestral lands of the IPs. Recently, I saw an old friend in Rio Tuba who was one of those Chieftains who had been validated by the government. He told me that those government officials came to his area with the mining company and they tried to pay him and the tribal council to conduct mining there. They refused and said it would be bad for them and the health of their children. But sad to say, he was denounced by the NCIP later and now a new Chieftain has been sworn in—one who has let the mining companies in. This is very common and it is how those mining companies persuaded so many villages to accept mining.

To some extent, in the field of local governance, it was difficult to comprehend or untangle motivations and to separate truth from lies, rumour from fact. I do not mean to say that all local government officials professed the views I have expressed here, nor consistently acted in ways that I have described. What I can say is that malaria appeared deeply embroiled in local politics one way or another and that this politicisation was particularly acute during election season. For example, in the lead up to the Mayoral election in May 2013, in which the incumbent Mayor's wife was running for the position, campaigning was prolific and malaria took centre stage. Health leaders were enthusiastically asked to report figures to local politicians who were keen to hear about and disseminate how malaria targets had been met and elimination almost achieved to prospective voters. I attended events where *Barangay* Health workers (BHWs) were solicited to hold awareness campaigns and spread messages of success particularly relating to the inroads made with malaria under the Mayor that were then promised to be continued under his wife's governance. One or two cautiously complained to me about having their efforts diverted to these kinds of campaigning operations, leaving them less time to conduct their 'real' health duties. Worse, casual workers told me that they felt they were endorsed for their positions specifically due to their assumed political allegiance, putting them in an especially insecure position in the lead up to and following elections. In order to 'volunteer' for the role of BHW for example, applicants needed only to informally consult *Barangay* Captains in order to be endorsed and have their papers signed off. As well as anxiety over job security, many were concerned for their own safety and that of their families. For example, one BHW told me she felt very scared during the election because she supported the opposition Mayoral candidate. She was so nervous when she was conducting her duties that she avoided some households and areas, despite knowing that people there might have needed minor medical attention. She was very careful about who she discussed politics with in case the Mayor's 'men were watching her' as she put it. Following the election of the Mayor's wife, she lost her job and felt sure that it was for these political reasons. For staff on a permanent contract, the situation was slightly better; however, senior and permanent workers too worried about being 'watched' or 'listened to' were unwilling to discuss politics in the open.

In the arena of municipal governance, malaria was therefore largely framed and dealt with as health problem of the 'past', under control because of leader's success at pushing forth with 'development'. As well as economic gain, in part, working towards 'good health' also justified agricultural development, mining and tourism on Indigenous lands. While these changes were certainly welcomed by some in Pälawan communities due to the employment, security and benefits they said they enjoyed as a result, for others, changes to the land not only disenfranchised them further but actually exacerbated their health problems. Many older Pälawan, for example, told me that '*malarya*' was a 'modern' problem—brought to the islands by migrants working in agroforestry and mining, and aggravated by population increase and more sedentary living arrangements. 'We have always had fever from *bati* here but now; we also get *malarya*. It looks almost the same but it is a new problem, brought from the outside. The way we live now causes it to come out', one lady told me. Health staff too reported that the recent increase in a number of health conditions including respiratory infections, skin conditions, accidents and vector-borne diseases such as malaria and dengue fever were a direct result of land-use changes. In the case of malaria, plantations and mining activity increased pools of stagnant water available for mosquitoes to breed and transmission was intensified due to migration, movement and population density. In fact, health staff were so sure that mining in particular was the cause of so many illnesses they were seeing, that they were heavily lobbying both the local government and mining companies to extend their CSR activities to all *barangays* in Bataraza, beyond the 11

Impact Areas south of the area of Tarusan as was then the case. In this way, malaria was being co-opted into health workers and *panglima's* polit-ical strategies to resist encroachment on their land and retain some of the power that had been stripped from their neighbours. As one senior health worker told me:

> I am very upset that their activities such as providing health care and schooling and homes is only for some here who were only willing to par-ticipate when bribed. How can those companies say that the effects of their mining stops at the line of Tarusan? Can they control the effect on the land and the air and the sea exactly to that point? Of course, the other 11 *baran-gays* beyond that point are affected and of course this is one of the main reasons why malaria and dengue are increasing. I have the figures here and can show them that rates are going up. So, me and some other *panglimas* are using this to challenge mining but also convince them to provide ser-vices for health in *all* those other places beyond Tarusan even if they don't accept mining. The companies can deny these effects but we are also talk-ing to the Mayor and all the *Barangay* Captains. They cannot ignore the figures.

Conclusion

As local government leaders enacted their agendas to sustainably develop land and the people who inhabited it in Bataraza, the malaria that health workers and community members claimed emerged as a direct result was dismissed or denied outright as being an issue. In addition to malaria, people argued that changes to the landscape were also causing 'old' causes of fever to increase. As explained in more detail in Chap. 5, *diwata*, or spirits who live within, own and master the seas, ground, forests, moun-tains, animals and plants, were increasingly being agitated by human activity. When spirit homes that are mainly located in the forests were disturbed, *bati* (Tagalog) emerged, manifesting in different ways but usu-ally as fever, chilling, sweating, body pain, rashes, insomnia or stiffness. For example, in a similar vein to Nernas above, Tirungan told me, 'there is more *bati* now because business people come and cut down those big trees or places where the *diwata* live to build plantations or do mining. But we too, we have less space to build our houses or *kaingin* so of course we are also disturbing them but we have nowhere else to go anymore now that we are losing our land.' Palawan and Bataraza more specifically offer a range of economic opportunities for those that venture there but this comes at a high price for its Indigenous People. In the face of such misfortune and illness, people can turn to a range of professionals to help treat their ailments, and for some Pälawan healers, just like the *panglimas* who entangle malaria in their efforts to resist appropriation, malaria is harnessed by these actors as a source of professional power. It is to these members of the community that I turn in the next chapter.

References

Balana, C. D. (2011). Palawan tribal folk hit use of fake leaders. *Philippine Daily Inquirer*.

Conklin, H. C. (1957). *Hanunóo agriculture: A report on an integral system of shifting cultivation in the Philippines*. Food and Agriculture Organization.

Conklin, H. C. (1961). The study of shifting cultivation. *Current Anthropology, 2*(1), 27–61.

Cramb, R. A., Colfer, C. J. P., Dressler, W., Laungaramsri, P., Le, Q. T., Mulyoutami, E., … Wadley, R. L. (2009). Swidden transformations and rural livelihoods in Southeast Asia. *Human Ecology, 37*(3), 323–346.

Dressler, W. H. (2005). Disentangling Tagbanua lifeways, Swidden and conservation on Palawan Island. *Human Ecology Review, 12*(1).

Dressler, W. H. (2006). Co-opting conservation: Migrant resource control and access to national park management in the Philippine Uplands. *Development and Change, 37*(2), 401–426.

Dressler, W. H. (2009). Old thoughts in new ideas: State conservation measures, development and livelihood on Palawan Island.

Dressler, W. H. (2014). Green governmentality and swidden decline on Palawan Island. *Transactions – Institute of British Geographers (1965), 39*(2), 250–264.

Dressler, W. H. (2019). Governed from above, below and dammed in between: The biopolitics of (un)making life and livelihood in the Philippine uplands. *Political Geography, 73*, 123–137.

Dressler, W. H., McDermott, M., Smith, W., & Pulhin, J. (2012). REDD policy impacts on indigenous property rights regimes on Palawan Island, the Philippines. *Human Ecology, 40*(5), 679–691.

Dressler, W. H., & Pulhin, J. (2010). The shifting ground of swidden agriculture on Palawan Island, the Philippines. *Agric Hum Values, 27*(4), 445–459.

Dressler, W. H., & Roth, R. (2011). The good, the bad, and the contradictory: Neoliberal conservation governance in rural Southeast Asia. *World Development, 39*(5), 851–862.

Dressler, W. H., Smith, W., Kull, C. A., Carmenta, R., & Pulhin, J. M. (2020). Recalibrating burdens of blame: Anti-swidden politics and green governance in the Philippine Uplands. *Geoforum, 124*, 348–359.

Dressler, W. H., Smith, W., & Montefrio, M. J. F. (2018). Ungovernable? The vital natures of swidden assemblages in an upland frontier. *Journal of Rural Studies, 61*, 343–354.

Dressler, W. H., Wilson, D., Clendenning, J., Cramb, R., Keenan, R., Mahanty, S., … Lasco, R. D. (2017). The impact of Swidden decline on livelihoods and ecosystem services in Southeast Asia: A review of the evidence from 1990 to 2015. *Ambio, 46*(3), 291–310.

Eder, J. F. (1987). *On the road to tribal extinction: depopulation, deculturation, and adaptive well-being among the Batak of the Philippines / James F. Eder.* University of California Press.

Eder, J. F. (1997). *Batak Resource Management, Belief, Knowledge and Practices.* Gland.

Eder, J. F., & Fernandez, J. (1996). *Palawan at the crossroads: Development and environment on a Philippine frontier.* Ateneo de Manila University Press.

Espino, F., Beltran, M., & Carisma, B. (2004). Malaria control through municipalities in the Philippines: Struggling with the mandate of decentralized health programme management. *International Journal of Health Planning and Management, 19*, S155–S166.

Larsen, R. K., Dimaano, F., & Pido, M. D. (2014). *The emerging oil palm agro-industry in Palawan, the Philippines: Livelihoods, environment and corporate accountability.* Stockholm Environment Institute.

Linn, B. M. (2000). *The Philippine War, 1899–1902.* University Press of Kansas.

Macdonald, C. J.-H. (2007). *Uncultural behavior, an anthropological investigation of suicide in the southern Philippines.* University of Hawai'i Press.

Magno, C., & Gatmaytan, D. B. (2013). *Free prior and informed consent in the Philippines: Regulations and realities.* Routledge.

Matsumoto-Takahashi, E. L. A., Tongol-Rivera, P., Villacorte, E. A., Angluben, R. U., Jimba, M., & Kano, S. (2018). Bottom-up approach to strengthen community-based malaria control strategy from community health workers' perceptions of their past, present, and future: a qualitative study in Palawan, Philippines. *Tropical Medicine and Health, 46*, 24–24.

Montefrio, M. J. F. (2017). Land control dynamics and social-ecological transformations in upland Philippines. *The Journal of Peasant Studies, 44*(4), 796–816.

Novellino, D. (2000a). Forest conservation in Palawan. *Philippine Studies, 48*(3), 347–372.

Novellino, D. (2000b). Recognition of ancestral domain claims on Palawan island, the Philippines: Is there a future? *Land reform: Land Settlement and Cooperatives, 1*, 57–72.

Novellino, D. (2000c). Recognition of ancestral domain claims on Palawan island, the Philippines: Is there a future? *Land Reform. Land Settlement and Cooperatives, 2000*(1), 56–72.

Novellino, D., & Dressler, W. H. (2009). The role of "Hybrid" NGOs in the conservation and development of Palawan Island, The Philippines. *Society & Natural Resources, 23*(2), 165–180.

Pulhin, J. M., & Dressler, W. H. (2009). People, power and timber: The politics of community-based forest management. *Journal of Environmental Management, 91*(1), 206–214.

Pulhin, J. M., & Pulhin, P. M. (2003). Community-based forest management in the Philippines: Retrospect and prospects. In M. Inoue & H. Isozaki (Eds.), *People and forest – Policy and local reality in Southeast Asia, the Russian far East, and Japan* (pp. 139–156). Springer Netherlands.

Ramos, B. (2013). Protecting Palawan. *The Philippine Star.*

Sandalo, R., & Baltazar, T. (1997). *The Palawan biosphere reserve: Philippines.* UNESCO.

Scott, G. A. J. (1979). The evolution of the socio-economic approach to forest occupancy (Kaingin) management in the Philippines. *Philippine Geographical Journal, 23*(2), 58–73.

Smith, W. (2018). Weather from incest: The politics of indigenous climate change knowledge on Palawan Island, the Philippines. *The Australian Journal of Anthropology, 29*(3), 265–281.

Smith, W. (2020). *Mountains of blame climate and culpability in the Philippine Uplands / Will Smith.* Seattle University of Washington Press.

Smith, W., & Dressler, W. H. (2017). Rooted in place? The coproduction of knowledge and space in agroforestry assemblages. *Annals of the American Association of Geographers, 107*(4), 897–914.

Suarez, R. K., & Sajise, E. J. (2010). Deforestation, Swidden agriculture and Philippine biodiversity. *Philippine Science Letters, 3*(1).

The Philippine Star. (2013). 3 dead is Palawan ambush. *The Philippine Star.*

Theriault, N. (2017). A forest of dreams: Ontological multiplicity and the fantasies of environmental government in the Philippines. *Political Geography, 58,* 114–127.

5

Practices of Professionalisation

Introduction

Remedios asks to meet in private. He tells me it is because he does not want to reveal his ability in healing to anyone else lest it diminishes. If others were to hear of how he came to be a *balyan* (healer), he may no longer be able to help them. When we are together, he pulls two smooth, shiny stones out his pocket that are wrapped in a frayed blue handkerchief. One is large and black and the other small and grey. He rubs them in the palm of his hand as he tells me they are *anting-anting* (charms/amulets) given to him by his *kagurangurangan* (ancestors) on his mother's side who were also *balyan*. He can prove to me they are *anting-anting* and not just normal stones because despite what I might expect, they float in water rather than sink as ordinary stones would. In front of him is a small china bowl filled with water that he lowers the objects into. Sure enough, they float on the surface. And sure enough, this defies my expectations. As he lifts the *anting-anting* out of the bowl, he mutters words under his breath that I cannot make out. 'I am asking for forgiveness from the *diwata* (spirits) for talking to you about this but it's OK because you have become like my child' he says. Remedios recounts the story of how he came to be a *balyan* after forming a 'special' relationship with a particular *diwata* in his dreams and how, as part of treatment for his patients, the *diwata* shows him which plants to use. When he sleeps, his *diwata* companion 'shows' him the way. In the case of *malarya* (Tagalog for malaria, but also denoting a broader illness category than biomedical conception) that 'comes up' when people are weak or suddenly exposed to cold after being warm (*pasma*), he can make up small pouches filled with seven kinds of plants. Once he collects the plants from the forest, he keeps them in his woven *tingkep* (lidded basket) that was also given to him by his *kagurangurangan*. Plants must be stored in the *tingkep* and kept hidden from his patients—his *anting-anting*, the plants and the *tingkep* (woven from bamboo with a rattan frame) are all imbued with g*inawa* (life force) he tells me. It is the *ginawa* that heals, not me and that comes ultimately from *Ampu* (the ultimate 'creator', 'owner' or 'master'). 'You see, when you are *keseud* (wise or expert), you must not share what you know with others in detail. The ability to see what makes people sick and what you need for healing is special for you only from *Ampu*—to share it lessens it.'

In this chapter, I turn my focus to some of the healers who diagnosed and treated malaria (or *malarya*) in Bataraza in order to show how their practice was bound up with their own (un)conscious strategies to build and retain their 'ability' as 'experts', as Remedios put it, or as legitimate professionals (Last & Chavunduka, 1986). Here, I show how healers from different 'traditions' did not necessarily differ in terms of their 'perceptions' of what malaria/*malarya* was (or wasn't), nor did they necessarily always engage in strikingly different practices in relation to diagnosing or treating it and similar illnesses. Rather, across all healers, I saw distinct parallels in the way that malaria/*malarya* and febrile illness was consistently conceived of and dealt with, alongside shared practices of professionalisation. Within the field of healing, people such as Remedios worked to distinguish themselves, not so much from each other but from their patients, through learning and enacting specific knowledge and training that established them as 'experts'. I show how four other healers—a Pälawan *balayan*, a *manghihilot* (bone setter), a *Barangay* Health Worker (BHW) and a pharmacist—also underwent extensive training following a 'calling' into their respective professions. They described how the esoteric knowledge and practices that they acquired gave them all access to an ability their patients did not possess—the power to 'see' the 'unseen' circumstances that resulted in sickness. All the healers that I encountered used potent objects for diagnosis and treatment in their practice, and the way in which these worked was somewhat intentionally shrouded from patients (as well as from me) by a degree of mystery. As a result, the malaria/*malarya* of professionalisation was a 'hidden' entity (expressed as 'things', 'dirt' or 'parasites') located inside bodies that needed to be 'uncovered' and dealt with by experts using their specific knowledge, objects and networks (in both the human and spirit realm). In the field of healing, malaria appeared to be co-opted into strategies of legitimisation on the part of healers who were fighting to uphold their status in a therapeutic landscape where multiple treatment options were available to patients.

Bataraza's Therapeutic Landscape

As described so far in this book, malaria attracted a lot of attention and action in Bataraza. Unsurprisingly, a range of healers claimed specific expertise in dealing with it or with sicknesses that seemed very similar to it. Building on anthropological concepts such as 'medicoscapes' (Hörbst & Wolf, 2014) and 'medical landscapes' (Hsu, 2008), I follow a number of authors in the fields of health geography and medical anthropology in using the term 'therapeutic landscape' (Gesler, 1992) to describe 'zone[s] of experience and meaning' (Wilson, 2003, p. 84) where multiple therapeutic possibilities are available, experienced, understood and enacted through practice by the population that provide and use them (Hampshire et al., 2011; Leach et al., 2008). In other words, the term refers to the places (both utilitarian and symbolic/interpretive) in which people take action to deal with sickness (Martin et al., 2015). Through recourse to the notion of landscapes, these approaches highlight the more fluid and ephemeral contours and features of different locales where various configurations of people, objects, ideas and practices come together in overlapping and complex ways that defy typologising within strict material-spatial bounds (Hsu, 2008). As Smyth (2005) pointed out, landscapes are also inherently open to scrutiny through a political-economic lens as unequal power relations and forces such as wealth inequity and globalisation (Hörbst & Wolf, 2014) influence their definition, shape and use—specifically how therapy or healing is defined, what is needed for it to take place, who is able to provide it and who has access to it (and by extension, who is excluded from these processes). In Bataraza, the therapeutic landscape was one in which a number of healers operated and competed for legitimacy, implicating disease as they did so. However, the sense of competition appeared to be less present among these healers as a group of peers but more pronounced in relation to defining their expert status relative to the patients they served.

In terms of what form healers' practices took at the time of fieldwork, government expenditure on 'formal healthcare', grounded in biomedical ideas, constituted 4.7% (in 2014) of Gross Domestic Product (GDP) which was less than the World Health Organization's recommendation of 5% (Mendoza, 2009) at the time. As such, the 'informal sector', grounded in traditional, complementary and alternative medicinal (TCAM) played a much more significant role in creating employment, producing goods and services and augmenting income (ibid.). In many areas of the country, 'informal' health practitioners were the main provider of healthcare (Tan, 2008). Staggeringly, while one 'informal' professional was available for every 300 Filipinos, only one 'formal' carer was available for every 26,000 (Mendoza, 2009, p. 334). In recognition of the fact that the 'hidden enterprise' of TCAM could both meet the needs of a population 'tired of conventional medicine' (ibid., p. 335) and drive economic growth, the Philippine government took steps to integrate TCAM within the formal economy. In 1997 the Traditional and Alternative Medicine Act (TAMA) was passed. As Mendoza (2009) explains, it was met with a high degree of resistance from medical groups, pharmaceutical companies and scientific organisations, worried about quality control, safety and efficacy and also suspicious that the government was motivated to promote TCAM due to the lucrative potentiality of foreign medical tourism. Nevertheless, the Philippine Institute of Traditional and Alternative Health Care was established within the Department of Health and was tasked with promoting and delivering TCAM products, services, modalities and technologies that had been 'proven' safe, effective, affordable in line with government standards as well as to provide research and skills training in alternative healing methods (ibid.).

While distinguishing provision of care according to 'types' of 'system' or 'traditions' in this way has practical and analytical utility, it invites a tendency to pit systems such as biomedical and folk; modern and traditional; formal and informal and public and private against each other as mutually exclusive, bounded categories that are necessarily antagonistic in practice. This creates an illusion of ontological difference between various groups that corresponds with discernible differences in both beliefs and practice among healers (as well as patients), in turn implying a degree of divergence and conflict between them. However, it ignores the role that unequal power relations play in influencing which systems 'dominate', 'colonize' or even 'co-opt' others for strategic reasons (Brodwin, 1996; Hampshire & Owusu, 2013). Much anthropological work has also crucially highlighted how such categorisations ignore the diversity and hybridity (Hsu, 2008; Parkin, 2013) that often exists in each context and overlooks the ability that actors have to intentionally ignore, transcend or even dissolve boundaries as much as they are able to reinforce them (Marsland, 2007). I illustrated this to some extent in Chap. 3 where I discussed how health leaders in Bataraza intentionally adopted biomedical perspectives and practices (and thereby reinforced the categorical boundaries of this system) despite the 'interferences' that existed for their own strategic reasons. In the field of healing that I describe here, while there were some similar distinctions enacted between experts from different 'traditions' in an effort to maintain boundaries, the reverse was also true and borderlines appeared more blurred in other cases. Much like health leaders, healers' practices were equally motivated by their own strategic reasons rather than simply being a mere product of their distinct roles defined in specific fields (Bourdieu, 1977). I demonstrate this by describing how the practices of healers were not necessarily aligned with clearly bounded, pre-existing, internally coherent 'systems' (Last, 1981). Instead, in a diverse but competitive therapeutic landscape, there was similarity in that their practices were (un)consciously motivated by expert's desires to carve themselves out as professionals first and foremost who could identify, and extract, sickness in bodies.

Sario, the *Balyan*

Wow! So many things happened. I was lying down and snakes were there, so those are like temptations, like a test. On the fifth night, I was starving and yet no answer for my prayers, but on the sixth night I began to hear some strange sounds like the sound of metal jangling and on the seventh night in the morning, early at dawn, there was a small boy in front of me who asked me 'What do you want? Why are you here?' So, I said, 'I want the ability to heal sick people. I want you to help me.' He said 'OK, wait until tomorrow'. The next day [day seven], I heard a rushing wind, and then later I saw a big man in front of me who was seven foot wide … and he said 'What do you want?'. I said, 'I want the ability to heal sick people' … and so the man said, 'OK, I'll give you what you want' and he gave me a stone—an *anting-anting*. … Then, from that time on, I began to have *kependeyan* (supernatural/miraculous powers) in my life. … If I am holding the *anting-anting* and I put it to my ears, I can hear *diwata* talking, even from the mountains—I can hear what the *diwata* are saying … they show me how to heal people. That is how I became a *balyan*.

Sario was a middle-aged man living with his wife Pina and her relatives in a small upland community in line with Pälawan conventions for matrilocal residence whereby women, namely sisters, join the community together and in-marrying men are said to 'stick' (-*pikit*) to their high status, wife-giving, fathers-in-law (Macdonald, 2007). Sario had a cautious, reflective and modest demeanour about him—characteristics that I found to be common among *balyan* that I met. He came from a line of *balyan* and had therefore acquired some of his knowledge and skills about how to heal from his *kagurangurangan*. He told me that although he wanted to be practicing in the community since a young age in order to follow in their footsteps, he had not had a 'calling' from a *diwata* guide to do so until much later in his adult life. One night, a figure that he thought was his deceased uncle (also a *balyan*) appeared to him in a dream and instructed him to go to a nearby cemetery, dig a hole and wait in it for seven days and seven nights with no food and to pray for some kind of 'power'. The first time he did this he saw some *diwata* in his dreams but nothing more came of this experience. He repeated the exercise some months later, and as he described above, this time, he had success. Now, not only did he possess an *anting-anting* but had a relationship with specific *diwata* who helped him diagnose and treat various ailments. I did not meet or hear of any female *balyan* but other practitioners that I encountered reported a similar 'calling' into the profession. In dreams or even death-like experiences, these men met *diwata* who had the capacity to appear as 'people' or 'humans' (*taqaw*), often in the form of a child or an elderly person. These figures enquired after them and offered help. All *balyan* reported having subsequent life-long links with particular *diwata*, some describing it as a kind of sibling relationship. Apart from this initial calling where some expertise was imparted, training was a long-term and practical endeavour and many *balyan* underwent a period of apprenticeship from relatives or close friends. There was a sense that a master would only agree to share his knowledge with those who possessed the 'right' kind of personality and displayed characteristics such as sincerity, modesty and loyalty, particularly through imitating the teacher's practices. For example, I met a master who explained that his apprentice 'must use the things that I use and do as I do'. His apprentice corroborated the importance of mimetic learning:

> The student has to be interested and show he is keen and committed to learn. The teacher has to see first his sincerity and loyalty to him as a teacher as if he is your father and you his son and then if he sees these good qualities, he will teach him to do as he does.

As Novellino (2001) argued, the knowledge and skill that *balyan* acquired was not simply the expression of a transcendental entity. Rather, *balyan* had to engage as active agents in the real-world task of learning their craft. He goes on to suggest this can traced back to Pälawan origin myths in which the separation of humans from *diwata* led to a transition from an age of abundance to an age of scarcity in which humans also acquired their immortality. As a result, people quite literally had to learn for themselves how to survive within the universe.

While Sario was reluctant to tell me the precise details of his interactions with *diwata* and the specific knowledge they imparted to him (for similar reasons to Remedios), he was keen to show me his practice. Thanks to what Sario described as *kependeyan*, he was able to 'see' (*memiriq*) and treat a range of sicknesses. In terms of diagnostics, I watched how he employed a mixture of bodily practice and the application of diagnostic tools to help him discover what he described as the 'hidden' reasons behind illness. When patients would come to him, he would spend some time observing them before saying or doing much himself. He explained that when he met a patient, he was looking for something specific. If he could see tiny worm-like coils coming out of their eyes and smoke coming out of their noses, then he knew they were suffering from sicknesses that were better treated in the Rural Health Clinic (RHU). This 'first step' as he called it was crucial as it allowed him to quickly triage patients, sending them to the Municipal Health Officer in the town where appropriate. This was the case for *malarya* as, according to him, this 'modern' illness was from 'things in the body' that he 'could not see' and therefore could not treat. 'How do people get *malarya*?' I asked him, 'I do not know. All I know is the people from the RHU came here and told us, there is this sickness called *malarya* inside the body and you must go to the clinic if you have it inside you—only they can see it.' Sario reported that he had many patients come to him over the years who were suffering from this illness that he now could put a name to. Sario saw the signs described above and referred patients on to other specialists who had the ability to see, and therefore treat, this particular ailment.

However, many patients came to Sario with afflictions that looked very similar to what the RHU staff had talked about in relation to *malarya*: fever, chills, headaches, fatigue and so on. However, a lack of the visual signs described above told him they were suffering from 'old' sicknesses that, due to his specific training, he had gained a reputation for being able to deal with. The 'second step' in these cases was to find the specific circumstances that led to the patient's illness. To do this, Sario would first use his index and middle fingers to feel the patient's pulse, closing his eyes and silently calling upon the *diwata* with whom he had established a relationship with to assist him in his diagnosis. As he explained, when people were sick, blockages could be felt under the skin, helping him to determine the aetiology of illness as described in more detail below. In addition, he used a *tari-tari*. This diagnostic tool was a hollow bamboo stick with honeybee wax at one end from which a piece of *rocoroco*

(*Ocimum sanctum* L. or Holy basil) was attached. As Novellino (2002) points out, different varieties of honeybees occupy a particularly important place in Pälawan cosmology given their ability to move between different levels of the universe (which are described in more detail below). The collection of *mugdung* (hives) for honey and wax such as that on Sario's *tari-tari* was a risky and skilled business. For *balyan* like him, small varieties of bee called *kätih kätih* in Palawano—which derives from the word *kätiän*: to attract or charm—are particularly important for healing purposes despite only producing negligible amounts of honey. As well as possessing an 'attractive' power in themselves, bees are in turn drawn to fragrant flowering plants such as *rocoroco* which has an herbaceous, musky, minty aroma—the very aroma that wafted in my direction as Sario proudly showed me his *tari-tari*. Sario's diagnostic tool was personal and specific to him—it was made by his father (also a *balyan*) and he inherited it from him after his death. The *tari-tari* was the same length as the span of Sario's hand but became longer or shorter to respectively confirm or refute the questions that he asked. Sario would ask each question to *diwata* (e.g., about the source of the illness or appropriate plants for treatment) three times and had to receive the same answer (indicated through the changing length of the *tari-tari*) all three times to ensure the answer was validated.

As well as consulting *diwata*, Sario also engaged in conversation with his patients. For him, discovering the origins of sickness was a practical endeavour that involved searching for answers through interaction with both unseen entities and human ones. For example, one evening a man came to see Sario with fever and feelings of weakness. The patient's father told Sario that he believed his son was suffering from *pintas* (Tagalog for a criticism, fault-finding or 'evil' words). Sario was able to confirm this was indeed the reason behind the man's fever through feeling his pulse and using his *tari-tari*. From the patient's narrative he was able to piece together the specifics—that the negative words had been spoken by a scorned lover with a 'sharp tongue' but it was due to his expertise that he could confirm the family's suspicions and, crucially, treat the illness. He explained the diagnostic process as he felt the man's pulse:

[I touch] this portion of the wrist [indicates part of the wrist below the thumb above the radius]. If it's *pintas* then it feels very hard and it is a human who brought the sickness. But in this portion [indicating part of the wrist below the little finger and above the ulna], if it has a very strong pulse that means they have a sickness from the forest, or mountains or bad *diwata*.

In order to consult with various *diwata* in his dreams for further guidance about treatment, Sario invited the patient to stay overnight in his house and instructed him to take a warm bath very early the next morning in order to release the blockage causing the fever and help 'send the curse back to the person who gave it to him'. He also gave him what he called a *pananga* which is an example of *panulak* (Tagalog for 'to push' intimating a repellent that can also be in a drink form) to wear once he had left. This small cloth pouch, which was sewn by Sario's wife Pina, contained seven specific medicinal plants and roots, the contents of which were revealed to Sario by *diwata* in his dream the proceeding night. As he prepared the plants, Sario directed his *tawar* (incantations) to the *diwata* that were 'masters' of the plants he was using. If tied round the waist of the patient using string, the *panulak* would also help reverse the negative words by 'pushing them back' and protecting the patient against further attacks. I was not surprised that Sario did not reveal the specifics of this treatment to me or his patients. For the Pälawan I met, although *adat pagbagi* (sharing) and *tabang* (mutual help) were crucial to the maintenance of social relations and very strong forces in regulating everyday life, as I describe in Chap. 6, these sentiments did not pervade the realm of healing in the same way. The reason given for the selective secrecy was the fear that the 'power' would diminish or lessen, as Remedios articulated, the more it was known about or talked about. In addition, pride and arrogance were seen as negative personality traits among many and highly offensive (Macdonald, 2007), whilst modesty, meekness and a mild demeanour were 'valued to a high degree' (ibid., p. 139). As one *balyan* elaborated:

> To make it a secret is the most important thing because the more it is secret, the more effective it is. If you boast about it then the power will

diminish. It comes back to the spirituality and the mentality of *Ampu*—to have patience and the attitude of *bahala-na* (Tagalog) or 'come what may'. For example, if somebody is sick over there, I cannot say 'oooh I know how to heal you—I know the healing practices, the herbal medicines for your sickness'. That is bad. That is bad … because you are boasting, being proud and lifting up yourself and anything you apply will have less power—it will not be effective. Come what may. That means that when a person comes then I'm not saying anything and later on, that person might say 'I want you to heal me'. If he insists that they want you to heal them then that is ok. You cannot announce it yourself in front of people but if they come to your house then it's ok because that means they are willing.

As well as illnesses brought on by human agents, Sario was also able to diagnose and treat those that occurred due to malevolent *diwata* but this process required more time and investigation. He told me that in Pälawan history, recounted by the *kagurangurangan*, *Ampu* 'wove' the world together in seven days. As well as crafting the visible environment and all living entities that dwelled within it, *Ampu* (who resided in seventh or most 'upper level' of the universe) also created a number of other *diwata*[1] who dwelled within lower levels but who mostly occupied (or were said to be masters of) the seas, ground, forests, mountains, animals, insects and plants that existed alongside humans in the 'middle level'. According to Revel (1990) and Novellino (2002), one *diwata*, *Upuq Mänungul*, was said by some to inhabit the lowest level (*basad*) and was charged with holding the universe from its base (*puqun*). By contrast, some *diwata* such as *Ampu at burak* (the master of flowers and bees) resided in an upper level closer to *Ampu* and could only be seen by *balyan* like Sario, hence the significance of flowers, flowering plants and bees in matters related to healing. Others that I spoke to made a distinction between harmful *diwata* that tended to live nearby, mainly in the forest or in *uma* (*swidden* fields), and friendly ones who lived high up in the mountains (I inferred they meant in places nearer to the elevated location of *Ampu*) although most people stressed that all *diwata* had the potential to be hostile or friendly depending on the situation/encounter and that these

---

[1] *Diwata* is a generic word for spirits used across the Philippines and Malaysia and derives from the Sanskrit *devata* meaning godhead or divinity (see Tan, 2008, p. 60).

were not necessarily mutually exclusive attributes. Human activity, especially in the forest or *uma*, could disturb or destroy places of residence, angering the *diwata* (e.g., through picking—or even complimenting the smell of—flowering plants reserved for bees, over-harvesting rice, trespassing in areas where harmful *diwata* lived etc.). This would result in *bati* (from *nabati* in Tagalog meaning to be greeted), or *salibegbeg/samban* (Palawano) whereby *diwata* would speak the name of the aggressor or brush past them, leading to symptoms including fever, chills, sweating, body ache, rashes, insomnia and the body becoming stiff or too strong to move. *Ampu* was also said to imbue all living plants, animals and humans with an essential source of life—*ginawa*, as Remedios mentioned above, which was crucial in healing processes. *Ginawa* was described an innate vital force, responsible for corporeal existence that stayed within the body (Tan, 2008) and connected people to an invisible network (Macdonald, 2007) as it was not just limited to human beings but also present in other entities such as plants, seeds, stones, animals, saliva and even words (whose potency therefore had the power to heal and harm). *Ginawa* was thus a source of health as well as potential source of illness as it could be manipulated through *pintas*. In addition, *Ampu* endowed humans with multiple *kurudwa*—souls that gave them their specific character as distinct from other living entities. The number and location of *kurudwa* differed between people I spoke to. However, there was consensus that the *kurudwa* located in the head was somehow different and superior to others. As one lady Lansi explained:

There are four *kurudwa*—one in the feet, hands, ears and head. [After death], the ones in the feet, hands and ears remain here on earth and can become ghosts but the *kurudwa* in the head goes to *Ampu*. When we die, it will stay above your head until the *balyan* cuts it and then it can go to *Ampu*. The *kurudwa* from the head is the only soul that is sensitive and can be easily offended. The result is that it can be removed from the body, even when you are still alive. We are all born with all these *kurudwa* but in children they are not yet securely attached and can come out easily, especially if they fall. That is why we take care with babies not to let them fall.

As Lansi intimates, unlike *ginawa*, people described how *kurudwa* were more like companions (dua/duwa meaning two in many Filipino languages) that had the ability to detach from the body and exist materially both spatially and temporally beyond a person's *bilug* (body) and even their lifetime. It was the detachable quality of the *kurudwa* that led to people becoming sick as their *compulsion* to wander off, mostly at night meant, meant they left a person lacking awareness and potentially in want (Tan, 2008), leaving the body vulnerable to negative forces. The *kurudwa* was linked by many to *nakem* (the mind) as the seat of 'understanding and awareness' (Tan, 2008) but not feelings and emotion which were restricted to the *atej* (liver) (Macdonald, 2007). Consequently, soul-loss came with a sense of unawareness described as feeling like being 'out of your mind' or 'unaware of your surroundings' and open to retribution from *diwata*. As such, *diwata* too were a source of sickness as well as healing. *Diwata* were thus both dangerous and protective and everyday life for all Pälawan was characterised by avoiding, assuaging and harnessing the unseen power that they lived alongside in order to avoid *sakit* (Tagalog for sickness/pain) within their own bodies, their communities and the cosmos as discussed in more detail in Chap. 6. *Balyan* therefore occupied a particular role in the community due to their 'expert' ability to see and negotiate with *diwata*, particularly ones such as *Ampu at burak* (the master of flowers and bees).

In order to treat sicknesses brought on by the actions of *diwata*, Sario had to enter *natutulog* (Tagalog for a sleeping state) so that his own *kurudwa* could leave his body to be replaced with *diwata* guides who were able to act as his double and to see and communicate with other invisible entities. It was this wandering quality of *kurudwa* that allowed people to dream (Macdonald, 2007) and for *balyan* such as Sario to heal. Sario would adorn a colourful *tadyung* (sarong) and *peleng* (cloth headband) with sprigs of *rocoroco* tucked into it. As well as being attracted by the fragrance, Sario explained that the vivid colours of his clothes allowed *diwata* to 'see' him and thus locate him. He would close his eyes, gently rock back and forth as he sat cross-legged on the floor and start to use *tawar*, inviting a double to enter him. Sario recounted how he would know a *diwata* had occupied his body because he would feel something like a wind enter him, followed by dizziness, but at the same time become unable to 'see' what was happening in the human world. I witnessed him suddenly jerk, bringing his body into a new sort of posture and attentiveness at the moment this seemed to happen. Sario would not be able to remember the details of what followed later on as in this state, the *diwata* would be his eyes, he explained due to feelings of unawareness brought on by such soul-loss. Once Sario's body had been taken over in this way, location and communication with other *diwata* was possible to assist with diagnosis and treatment. For example, one young man came to Sario complaining of fatigue and body ache, particularly in his back. Sario was able to use this diagnostic technique to determine the unseen agents behind the man's illness and told me:

> Some bad *diwata* had gone inside the back of this man to give him body pain. I can't remember who the *diwata* was because I was sleeping. Sad to say that the *diwata* in the mangroves got angry with this guy because he is always destroying the mangroves and I suspect that the *diwata* in the mangrove stabbed him using their *bolo* (knife) because he is not doing good in their place—maybe he is destroying their place.

In this case, malevolent *diwata* had entered the patient's body, displacing his *kurudwa*:

> When we are walking somewhere our own *kurudwa* are with us, but the other *diwata* [are more numerous] than people living here and these unseen *diwata* are able to grab hold of our *kurudwa*, if we do not have the defence, if we do not have protection then these bad *diwata* can enter us.

In order to treat this kind of soul-loss, Sario picked *rocoroco* tips which he waved in a circular motion over the patient along with *silad* (pom poms) made from Mangrove Fan Palm *(Licuala spinosa L.) accompanied by tawar to call helpful diwata to his aid. As he explains*:

> First, I use the *rocoroco* to remove the ailments like bad *diwata* … six times going round [in a circle] with the *rocoroco*. … Whatever *diwata* it is that makes the patient sick, it is attracted to and hangs on the *rocoroco*. Then, the seventh time, I will call the man's *kurudwa* to come back and when it is there, it also hangs onto the *rocoroco* so that I can then put it back inside

[using the *silad*]. I get the *silad* and do the same—round six times. ... The purpose of the *silad* is that when I am sleeping and holding the *silad*, any person who is suffering some kind of disease comes close to the *silad* then this *silad* will be the one to heal them. There is *ginawa* in that *silad*—it has a purpose of curing the disease because my power and the power of other *diwata* are going through that *silad*. Because my eyes are closed I cannot see anything, only the *silad* can see ... and it will take out the diseases that are there and return the lost *kurudwa* to the patient.

The ability to harness the power of *ginawa* in *anting-anting*, plants, *diwata* and people was therefore central to Sario's expertise. He, like most *balyan* I spoke to, gave rather ambiguous explanations for how exactly *ginawa* 'worked'. All he knew was that these methods brought success in alleviating pain and earned him a good reputation among his satisfied patients. In return for his services, the man brought Sario a chicken[2] as well as a few pesos, typical of the kind of remuneration I witnessed *balayan* receive.

Nicanor, the *Manghihilot*

Nicanor was an elderly man originally from Surigao which is located in the northeast coastal plain of the island of Mindanao. *His* father was sent to prison in Palawan and, upon his release, relocated his family to the island which is how Nicanor came to Bataraza. Like many Surigaonons, Nicanor told me he was Christian (likely Roman Catholic). Although the south of the archipelago had a long history of trade, exchange and habitation by Muslim traders, creating sizeable populations of and Tausug in Mindanao and Penimusan in Southern Palawan (Theriault, 2017), the Christian Surigaonon, who are part of the Visayan ethnolinguistic group, dominated in provinces such as Surigao. Nicanor also told me that he was a *manghihilot* (Tagalog for bone setter). By his own admission, he was renowned with patients coming to him from all over Palawan. He had never had a patient he could not treat except, sadly, himself. For the last

---

[2] Macdonald (2007) writes that in Pälawan cosmology, both human and *diwata* have animal substitutes. In the case of humans, chickens are a substitute for the human *kurudwa* and in the case of *diwata*, wild boar.

few years, he had been partially paralysed down one side of his lower body from an illness he could not fully explain nor relieve despite his best efforts. However, he professed himself lucky because his illness had not affected his hands, which for him were crucial to his practice as a *hilot* as they enabled him to be able to feel *naipit* (Tagalog for pinched or blocked), *ugat* (Tagalog for blood vessels) or *laman* (Tagalog for muscles) (see O'Malley, 2004). I had been told by many people to go and see Nicanor due to his reputation and expertise in treating malaria. I visited him one day and found him propping himself up on a pillow with one elbow, reclining on an otherwise bare wooden bench. Confined almost exclusively to this bed, he explained how his wife had moved it to the front of their two-roomed nipa house so that from this location, he could at least look out of the door and see the sky and flowers as he lay there for many hours of the day. I asked Nicanor how he became a *manghihilot*:

I am a twin. My twin was a snake[3] and when the moon was dark, she would take a bath and after ... she would become a woman. She is the one who taught me how to become a *manggagamot* (general Tagalog term for healer). ... She was long when she came out of the womb and when we were breastfeeding, I would take one breast and she would take the other but my mother would be out of consciousness because she was so afraid of the snake. She came out as a snake but we were attached by our umbilical cords. We lived together for 20 years. She loved to sleep under the *kulambo* (Tagalog for mosquito net) and when there were *lamok* (Tagalog for mosquitoes) around she would eat them. She lived in a separate room and in the evening time no one would enter her room because, at that time, she was a woman. She could understand words and would nod her head [when we spoke to her] ... she grew as long as the house and very high. All my cousins would come and ride on her and play with her ... we would ride on her back and then she would go faster and people would fall off [laughs]. She would be eating rice and when she finished her tail would tap meaning 'finished' and then me and my cousins would wash the plates. Then, one day, we fought about who came out the womb first so I hit her with a stick and she got angry and left. But I know she is still alive because we were attached by the umbilical cord so when one of us dies, the other will also die. I said I was the first born but she said 'no'. She said she saved me coming out from the womb. … When we were young, she would take me to the forest and bite the plants [used for healing] and while she was showing me, she would tap her tail on my forehead and say, 'you remember this' so that is how she taught me about being an *albularyo* (Tagalog for herbalist). I am also a *manghihilot* and I fix bones. She would wrap herself around me and crush all of my bones. Then she would tap me at the neck and all over and the bones would be healed. This is how I learnt how to do that kind of massage.

Nicanor was not alone in having special circumstances around his birth. Others that I met were born *suhi* (Tagalog for breeched). As one female *manghihilot* explained, the 'special ability to feel people's bones and blood vessels comes to those born in a special way'. Although Nicanor gained much of his early knowledge and skills from his twin sister, he explained that his decision to become a practicing *manghihilot* in the community was really down to his interactions with what he describes in English as the 'spirit' world. As Tan (2008) articulates, many Visayans, such as Nicanor, refer to these beings as *dili ingon nato* or the 'not like us' to denote their difference from regular humans, despite their humanly appearance, due to their disembodied state and capacity to bring on illness. Many years ago, when his son was sick, one such spirit, in the guise of an old man, came to him in a dream. He believed it was the ghost of one of his ancestors and he was able to tell Nicanor what plant could ease his child's pain. A succession of other dreams confirmed to Nicanor that he had a special 'gift' that allowed him to have a relationship with the invisible world. Ultimately, it was this 'calling to help the people', as he described it, that persuaded him to become a practicing *manghihilot*. While Nicanor was not officially registered by the Municipality as a government-approved *hilot*, many were. Training for *manghihilot*s (chiropractic practitioners) and *magpapaanaks* (birth attendants) began in 1954, and as such, registered practitioners were able to attend training courses to qualify as 'formal' professionals.

As I sat talking to Nicanor, a steady stream of patients came to see him with ailments ranging from body pain to fever. One Pälawan woman told me she had travelled for many hours because she had heard how good he was. When patients like her would enter, Nicanor would closely observe them whilst rubbing his hands with drops of oil infused with roasted and powdered tree bark that he kept in a bottle by his bed. After asking the patient to sit next to him, he would start to feel their pulse. Much like Sario, he would accompany this visual and tactile encounter with quiet whisperings, in his case to the 'Lord'. In between consultations he told me this combination of practices allowed him to locate the *sakit* in people's bodies, feel its specific origin within and invoke 'dream'-like visions to help 'reveal' the circumstances which led to the patient becoming sick at a particular time and/or location. He would simultaneously talk to patients who would sometimes also describe their feelings or conjecture over what they felt to be the conditions surrounding their illness. For example, some patients I witnessed told Nicanor they thought they were suffering from *bati* or *pintas*, similar to the ailments reported to Sario. However, Nicanor was adamant he did not base his diagnosis on what his patients told him as he was able to determine their illness, the circumstances that led to them and subsequently correct treatment via his own means. In all cases, massage and manipulation along with the use of different plant-infused oils worked to release blockages, create flow in the body and push the sickness 'out'. Indeed, all the patients that came to Nicanor when I was with him left relieved of the pain they came in with and were completely satisfied with his services. Most dropped a few pesos in his hand or offered baskets of bananas or pineapples in payment.

As well as ailments brought on by the actions of spirits and human agents such as *bati* and *pintas*, Nicanor specialised in treating sicknesses that came about due to disequilibrium in the body. In many cases, *lamig* (Tagalog for cold) was the culprit, entering bodily orifices as it clung to *hangin* (Tagalog for 'airs' or 'winds') or *pawis* (Tagalog for sweat). Once inside, through the pores, mouth or the nose for example, *lamig* could settle or rest in certain places causing *dugo* to thicken and *ugat* or *laman* to become stuck or swollen (O'Malley, 2004; Tan, 2008). It was this disruption to the flow of *dugo* which brought on the *sakit, pasma* (Tagalog for 'exposure' illness characterised by spasms, fever, fatigue, weakness and body ache) or even death. Nicanor described how *malarya* was a similar illness that arose due to what he described as 'too much' dirt entering the body from contaminated food, water or *lamok*, restricting *dugo* inside the body. For these patients, after feeling their pulse and using prayers to confirm their type and aetiology of illness, Nicanor looked at and felt the afflicted person's *baso-baso* (indicating abdomen), the swelling of which, along with fever, chills and body ache, were sure signs of *malarya*. He told me, 'the *baso-baso* feels hard because it becomes stuck from *malarya* and the person's lips will be white and pale as the flow of *dugo* is blocked. In this case it may be the most serious kind that affects the mind.' In these instances, Nicanor used a particular oil alongside the massage therapy that he administered to patient's abdomens, chest, back and head, working in a circular motion from the waist up in order to push the *pawis* out. He told me that fever and sweating arose in the body when *resistensiya* (Tagalog for resistance) was low and the body was weak. The base oil he used for *malarya* was extracted from specific coconuts that faced East, selected from trees that had only bore few fruits. Although he used to collect the coconuts himself, making sure never to drop them in the process in case it lessened their power, he had to rely on his eldest son to do this for him now. Once the coconut flesh had been shredded, mixed with water, heated and cooled, the oil could be harvested from the fruit pulp. It was then mixed with seven types of grass, root, bark and tree leaf which were all inhabited by various 'spirits'. Nicanor knew which plants were needed for this *malarya* oil because as he traversed the forest, the plants he needed would move or rustle, similar to how they did when his snake-sister would guide him. In his sister's absence, the spirits could now communicate with him directly he told me. Nicanor explained that it was the oil and its ingredients that contained the real 'power to heal' and not the massage/manipulation alone: 'without the oil, my hands are powerless'. So significant was this concoction that its exact contents were kept secret even from Nicanor's family. Like Sario, the number seven seemed to come up many times in Nicanor's practice—and seemed 'lucky' for many across the islands in general. *Balayan* and *hilots* told me that the reason *Ampu* or the Lord created the world in seven days was due to the fact it was '*hindi pares*' (not paired or equal in Tagalog). As an odd number, it would always 'have one over' evil or misfortune so to speak.

Although Nicanor used to treat many cases of *malarya*, he remarked how he had seen fewer and fewer of these patients in recent years acknowledging that they preferred to go and see 'modern' doctors in the RHU or hospital in Brooke's Point, because they too had strong and effective medicines. Consequently, if one of Nicanor's patients came to him with what he diagnosed as *malarya*, he would provide his own treatment but also advise them to go to these alternative healers if they were not better within a couple of days. Nevertheless, he maintained that as far as he knew this had never happened. He was confident that all of his patients had recovered from *malarya* after seeing him.

As such, similar to Sario, Nicanor did not seem to view himself in competition with other healthcare providers. While he was protective when it came to sharing the specific contents of his oil, there were other 'old' treatments, as he described them, that he was happy to talk openly about should anyone ask. In fact, over the years he reported that he had helped in the production of government-licenced tablets made from the plants he knew to be effective for illnesses such as fever and diarrhoea:

> The doctor asked me about remedies for diarrhoea. The herbal medicine I had for that is not so bitter and even the children can tolerate it. I told the doctors and we went to the forest together and I taught them. … That was seven years ago. The doctor injected in these plants and said 'yes it's true' and then they made tablets from the *sambong* (*Blumea balsamifera* L.) plant'.

Elyn, the *Barangay* Health Worker (BHW)

Armelyn, or Elyn for short as she liked to be called, was in her 40s when I met her and was married with children. Along with her family, she had moved to Bataraza over a decade ago from the north of Palawan and applied to become a BHW soon after. This decision was partly motivated by the practical need for her to earn some sort of income, no matter how modest, but also due to the fact that both her grandfather and her grandfather-in-law were *babalyan*—the Tagbanua equivalent of *balyan*. As such, she told me that she inherited a lot of knowledge of how to heal from both of them including the use of plants for medicinal purposes, making her an *albularyo* of sorts, she joked, similar to Sario and Nicanor. As my relationship with Elyn developed over many months, she also revealed to me that her grandfather had given her something else—what she described in English as a 'charm' before he died. Charms were not given lightly, she explained, and not just to anyone. Only people who possessed certain characteristics would inherit them. She knew of some *babalyan* who died without passing on their special objects. She therefore saw her decision to become a BHW as a 'natural' choice because of this ancestry and predisposition and described it as her 'calling'. In recent years she had also become one of the few malaria Rapid Diagnostic Test (RDT) specialists in Bataraza, servicing the *barangay* where she lived, which had seen sustained malaria transmission. For this role she had undergone specific training on malaria, its diagnosis and treatment. The content of this training was produced by organisations such as the World Health Organization and Department of Health and was largely bio-medical in nature. As such, Elyn explained to me in English that 'malaria is a disease caused by parasites that enter human blood through the bite of infected female mosquitoes'. In order to be sure someone had malaria 'they must be tested using an RDT or through examination of a blood film under a microscope so that the malaria can be seen'. In other conver-sations, Elyn told me about other knowledge that she had gained not from her formal BHW training but from her own lived experience. For example, according to her, symptoms may not necessarily manifest if you were strong, well-fed and healthy, even if the parasites were in your body. Rather, the likelihood of sickness 'coming out' was related to sudden changes in the weather or levels of hunger or energy. This knowledge that she gained was from her ancestors as well as from her own personal observations.

The malaria-specific training Elyn received as an RDT technician was supplementary to the basic training she had had to become a BHW. The Philippines was an early adopter of the community model for delivering primary care, launching the BHW programme in the early 1980s (Mallari et al., 2020). Each BHW undertook instruction from an accredited gov-ernment or Non-Government Organisation (NGO) in community health before being eligible to attend optional ongoing seminars and courses throughout their career, with some BHWs progressing onto acquiring official qualifications in nursing or midwifery. Again, the majority of the content of these courses was biomedical in nature and

Elyn recounted how at her week-long training programme run by the RHU, she was mostly told how to recognise the signs and symptoms of common childhood illness, warning signs in pregnant women or how to assess complaints such as aches, coughs, colds, high blood pressure, temperature and fever. More recently at other seminars she had attended, she noticed there had been some inclusion of information related to government-approved 'herbal' medicines that were now licenced for use by the Philippine Institute of Traditional and Alternative Health Care and available in tablet form in pharmacies. These included derivatives of plants she had already known about from her youth such as the *sambong* that Nicanor had mentioned for fever and diarrhoea and *lagundi* (*Vitex negundo L.*) for fever and respiratory conditions. Elyn continued her training by attending seminars or courses once or twice a year that she heard about through her superiors or colleagues, sometimes travelling as far as Puerto Princesa. She was extremely proud of this and articulated that she was always willing to attend more seminars because learning was a 'joy' to her. However, her ability to do so was largely dependent on whether or not she could afford the transport, even to those events located within Bataraza. The BHW position was after all 'voluntary'. The Benefits and Incentives Act of 1995 allowed for BHWs to receive a modest monthly honorarium to cover incidentals but this was determined by local governments and amounted to only 1000 PHS (£10).

In terms of the workload Elyn was expected to take on, although *Barangay* Health Stations (BHSs) were technically mandated to assign a maximum of 20 households to each BHW to cover, in Bataraza only one *barangay* had actually attained this ideal ratio. In reality, BHWs were responsible for anywhere between 20 and 300 households. Each week, they were instructed to spend one or two days working in the BHS or RHU, registering and triaging patients or performing tasks such as recording temperatures and blood pressure, or they were sent into the community to undertake specific activities such as distributing *filariasis* treatment or Vitamin A tablets. Outside of this, BHWs were then required to visit their households in order to check on patients and administer advice, or to suggest further courses of investigation or treatment for issues as far ranging as infectious diseases to maternal health. Accordingly, Elyn would try and visit as many of her designated 200 plus households as she could throughout the week. She explained that in reality it was difficult so she had developed a rotation system, only going to certain areas on certain days. That way, she had worked out she could get to each household roughly every four or five weeks. Elyn approached her work with efficiency and resolute commitment. She told me that she tried to complete her door-to-door calls in the mornings, often setting off as early as 5 or 6 am. In the afternoons, she would have to attend to her own household—cooking, cleaning, gardening, shopping or taking care of her children who were still young. It was a reminder that all the BHWs I met in Palawan were women and corroborated the view that although the country had a world-leading performance on several key indicators of gender equality, women's jobs were 'largely restricted to those considered as extensions of the mothering, caring and educating roles defined by a patriarchal worldview' (Mallari et al., 2020, p. 8). On the occasions when I accompanied her on her rounds, I was impressed by Elyn's energy, eagerness and fitness, but in all honesty, I struggled to keep pace. 'My father was very tall like me and Tagbanua are known for being strong in the legs', she shouted down to me as she confidently marched barefoot up the steep, rocky hillside, rain lashing down her impressively lean and muscular calves. I sensed that the phrase 'unlike you' was omitted from the end of her sentence as she sympathetically looked back at her by now bedraggled, out-of-breath companion, reduced to crawling on all fours through the liquid mud behind her.

To help assist her with her work, Elyn was given a thermometer, a sphygmomanometer to measure blood pressure and a bottle of paracetamol tablets from the RHU. BHWs on the whole were not licenced to perform diagnostics or administer treatments. Elyn, like many others, saw her role more as one of monitoring and supporting. She stated: 'I mainly ask to see who is sick and tell them to go to the health centre or remind them of our programmes'. However, as Elyn was also an RDT technician, she did have a wider remit and carried an extra bag containing bottles of alcohol, cotton swabs, packs of RDTs and first-line malaria treatments, namely Coartem[4] (to treat *Plasmodium falciparum*)

---

[4] Coartem is the company Novartis' brand name for their artemether-lumefantrine combination anti-malarial drug.

and Chloroquine (to treat *Plasmodium vivax*). This gave her the tools she needed to both diagnose and treat malaria in the field. Elyn also told me she knew about a number of other effective plant treatments for a range of illnesses including malaria. As such, she carried some of these with her from her own garden or picked some from those of her neighbours as she went about her rounds. 'Many of us know about these treatments from our ancestors. We grow these plants so we always have something nearby that we can use. It is for free and we can just share. It is alright to ask for these from your neighbours' she tells me as she brushes her hand across a fragrant *sambong* bush growing in her own garden alongside other medicinal plants, vegetables, fruits and flowers, notably her impressive array of colourful orchids. For malaria in particular, Elyn often prescribed the use of *sambong* to 'lower the fever and calm the head and stomach' in addition to the allopathic medicines that she had. She stressed however that the main 'treatment' she provided was encouraging people to go to the BHS or RHU to have further tests or medical attention. She showed me how to prepare *sambong*: 'first, you must pick the leaves like this, taking off the yellow flowers, then you soak the leaves in water and just leave them, do not pound too hard. After a while, when the water is dark in colour you can drink it. The taste is a *mapakla* (Tagalog for astringent) and a little cool.' Taking a sip myself, the concoction certainly hit bitter, acrid and camphorous notes and left a cool but dry sensation in my mouth. *Mapakla* was a word many used to describe the taste of various plants but 'astringent', 'bitter' or 'acrid' didn't seem to do it justice as a translation. Elyn described it perfectly when she said 'it is like the strings (or pith) inside a banana, especially when they are not yet ripe. It sticks in your mouth.' Elyn also showed me how the wet, warm leaves could then be applied to the forehead or stomach as a poultice to ease headache, diarrhoeal cramps or menstrual pain.

As well as testing and treating people in their own homes, Elyn told me that, every week, she also had number of patients come directly to her house presenting with a wide variety of symptoms but all reporting that they had malaria. Regardless of what her patients 'believed', Elyn always performed an RDT if they were suffering from any one of the symptoms she knew accompanied the presence of malaria; fever, chills, sweating, fatigue, headaches and/or body ache. As she explained:

Most of the people come to me and say that they have malaria but they don't know if they have really. In order to know you must test the blood. In the microscope you can see the parasites but in the RDT (Rapid Diagnostic Test), it shows up a line if there are parasites. Many people that come to see me know I am an expert in doing RDTs so they come here when they suspect they have malaria but in actual fact most of them do not because the numbers are very low here. They maybe have other things like dengue or UTI (Urinary Tract Infection). In that case, I will tell them they must go to the RHU to have the proper tests and treatment.

I was able to experience first-hand how Elyn performs such diagnostic tests. When we were out one day, I felt feverish and had a headache. As we sat in her friend's porch in the baking heat, she checked my temperature and blood pressure and, although both were within normal range, insisted she perform an RDT. She wiped my finger using a cotton swab soaked in alcohol; pricked my finger with a needle and used a plastic blood-transfer tube to take a drop of the blood and place it in the sample window on the test cassette. Buffer solution was added in the appropriate hole and then we waited for 15-20 minutes to see the result which, thankfully, was negative. Elyn suggested she look in the friend's garden to see if they had any plants that I could use to make a drink to immediately lessen my symptoms. As was consistent with her training, Elyn also advised me to go and have a blood smear test at the RHU. She explained that the parasite count in my blood could be too low to be detected by the RDT, saying 'it is only with a microscope that you can really "see" the parasites directly'.

Illaine, the Pharmacist

Like Elyn, Illaine was also in her 40s but unlike Elyn was petite at just 5 foot 3 inches. It was nevertheless impossible to miss Illaine with her beaming smile and infectious loud, cackle-like laugh. Although ethnically Ilocano, she was born in the neighbouring municipality of Brooke's Point as her parents had moved from Luzon to Palawan when she was young. Illaine was widowed and lived with her three children above the pharmacy she owned. She employed three younger women to work in her house and business. They stayed with her for much of the year, occupying a large attic room with panoramic views of the paddy fields and mountains that the pharmacy looked out on. I was lucky enough to live with Illaine and her household, taking her eldest son's room while he was away in college. Illaine studied Pharmacy in Manila and, after finishing her degree, moved back to Palawan. She married her husband in the early 1990s and then decided to move from Brooke's Point to Bataraza in order to open a pharmacy, seeing a gap in the market. She described how, at the time, there was no town centre in Bataraza or any decent infrastructure such as electricity or good roads. Only a few migrant 'lowlanders' like herself lived in the centre and the remaining largely forested land was mostly inhabited by Pälawan. The small pharmacy that she and her husband built and opened was the only one in the area, and when I met her, she remained the only officially licenced pharmacist in Bataraza. This was something Illaine was keen to remind her clients of in her friendly, informal manner and her certificates were proudly hung in full view on the walls of the pharmacy next to her collection of textbooks, which she regularly dipped into during consultations with customers. Together these acted as a badge of her professionalism, her equivalent *anting-anting* perhaps, and clearly set her apart from her less qualified or even illegal competitors. Illaine had invested many years in learning her profession and regularly corroborated, updated and refreshed her knowledge by referring to her books. Significantly, they were all in English and required a certain level of linguistic and scientific proficiency to render them comprehensible. This made the knowledge accessible to her in a way that it simply was not to the young women working for her, and certainly out of reach of most of her customers. Although I saw her impart some of what she knew to her staff regarding pharmacology, she was discriminating in terms of which staff she deemed most worthy. She described this as an issue of practicality—she did not have time to train all of them in-depth. However, her staff interpreted her actions differently. For example, Marisol confided in me that Illaine treated her 'better' than the others because theirs was a special relationship, more akin to mother and daughter than employer and employee:

She does not trust the others in the same way because of so many problems she had in the past. For example, most people worked here for the money and were not so interested to learn about the pharmacy from her. Some even stole from her. There have been many problems but I am like family to her. She gives us everything we need—a good salary and on top of that all the food we could ever want, a nice house to live in, she even pays the tricycle fare for us to go on trips or to see our family. Her children are like my siblings. She only teaches me. Maybe it is her plan that I can take over this pharmacy one day.

It was certainly true that I saw Illaine act differently towards Marisol, including encouraging her to talk with me in English, joking that it would help her understand her textbooks better.

Although her business had grown considerably over the years, and was now the main private provider of allopathic drugs, maintaining herself as a 'legitimate' practitioner was key to Illaine's success. A number of other much smaller licenced and unlicenced pharmacies had opened in the town as well as many *sari-sari* stores (road-side variety stores) selling a range of drugs, tablets, teas and creams. At the weekly market in the town centre, it was also possible to buy drugs, but many were said to be counterfeits coming mainly from Malaysia and China. Inspectors based in Manila would periodically come to Bataraza. Illaine told me that once they got to Puerto Princesa, shop owners would text each other to give prior warning that they were making their way south. The unlicenced shops would temporarily close down, cover up and their owners would leave town to avoid inspection. Illaine laughed as she proudly told me how, unlike them, she had no need for such deception. She actively welcomed the inspectors as she had 'nothing to hide', after all. All her drugs were 'legitimate' and of the 'highest quality'.

Having lived with Illaine for a year, I was able to learn a lot about her business as well as observe the way in which she and her staff dealt with customers. The majority came to her asking for allopathic medicines. In cases where customers asked for non-prescription drugs for 'mild conditions' including pain, coughing or 'flu, Illaine and her staff exchanged these with little discussion or further consultation with patients. However, many also asked for prescription-only drugs such as antibiotics or anti-malarials but without the necessary paperwork. Prescriptions were issued by Renya, the Municipal Health Officer stationed in the RHU, but, as described in Chap. 3, she was often absent or difficult to get an appointment with (being the only doctor). Although Danny, the Medical Technician, was also authorised to issue prescriptions, many people sought out the services of the pharmacy first. In these cases, Illaine would often enter into discussion with them, taking medical histories, sometimes referring to her books and attempting to make diagnoses and recommend the best course of treatment. In this way, she described to me that she felt she was always learning on the job and 'refreshing' her knowledge based on who came to her door. However, even when she knew and suggested to patients that they should have further tests done at the RHU to clarify the cause of their symptoms, Illaine, and her staff, would sometimes still sell patients prescription-only drugs. For example, although Illaine knew what the current first-line treatments for malaria were and that it was not advisable to give anti-malarials to people who had not had malaria confirmed by a diagnostic procedure (or the type distinguished) she sold them tablets of Chloroquine on occasion. As she explains:

If people come here with a fever, I tell them they should go see Danny first to get a test and see if they have parasites inside and then he will give them drugs for free if they are positive [for malaria] but even when people don't want to do that, I will still sell them anti-malarials sometimes if they ask for them. People are poor and cannot afford more than a few tablets. I tell them it is not effective to take only few [tablets] but what can they do? I feel sorry for them so I still sell them. Most people say they have malaria when they have any illness but it's always malaria malaria. They want Chloroquine even though it is only effective for *vivax*. I will still sell them Chloroquine as it is very cheap compared to other drugs—sometimes even just one or two tablets but I don't think they always have malaria—it's just to give them something, otherwise maybe they won't come back here to my store! [laughs]'

Illaine was not alone in this. All pharmacies, licenced or not, sold individual tablets including antibiotics and Chloroquine and it was very common to hear people report to staff in market stalls or *sari-sari* stores that they had *malarya* and needed a couple of tablets of Chloroquine. As well as allopathic drugs, Illaine also sold toiletries, confectionery and a wide range of 'herbal' medicines including licenced tablets and teas. Various kinds of incense and gem stones that had their roots in Chinese medicine had also become increasingly popular with customers in recent years. For example, one patient came to the pharmacy complaining that her young daughter was repeatedly falling sick with different afflictions including recurring fever. Although the young girl tended to get better after treatment with paracetamol or Chloroquine, the mother was concerned about the 'real' reasons for these frequent and recurring episodes. She wanted to ask Illaine, as a fellow Catholic, if she thought it could be that the child was being 'tormented by God's spirits'. Illaine told her that she thought it was possible but that she was not able to make such a diagnosis. Instead, she advised her to talk to her priest who would be better placed to help her on this particularity. However, Illaine did recommend that she buy a small red cloth envelope which, if pinned to the child's clothes, would act as a repellent to malevolent spirits. She also sold her some black coal which she advised to be burnt and carried around the whole house seven times in order to dispel any spirits which might be present in the house and afflicting the child with recurrent fever episodes. These were effective for dealing with spirits, Illaine told me, and tools that she had used in her own home to protect her family.

Conclusion

Sario, Nicanor, Elyn and Illaine all distinguished themselves (and were distinguished by others) as certain 'types' of healer: a *balyan*, *manghihilot*, *Barangay* Health Worker and a pharmacist. They were further categorised still, and ascribed labels such as 'formal' or 'informal', 'traditional' or 'biomedical', in certain circles. However, the knowledge and practices of all four healers did not necessarily fit into such discrete categories. Boundaries between them appeared somewhat more 'latticed' (Parkin, 1995) in nature. Securing legitimisation on the other hand was crucial to all and necessary in order that these practitioners attract patients. Professionalisation was in part conferred by their specific training. Many healers reported a hereditary background in therapeutics; however this was not a prerequisite as anyone, in theory, with enough training, both formal (through courses or apprenticeships) and informal (through hands-on practical experience), could become a practitioner. So long, it seems, as they possessed certain traits or characteristics. For *balyan* masters and Illaine, loyalty was key above all else. However, all reported a sort of 'calling' which convinced and encouraged them to work publicly and endowed them with the esoteric knowledge needed to uncover entities inside bodies afflicted *with* malaria/*malarya*. Success in doing so ensured the good reputation of all. Sario described 'things inside the body' that he could not see; Nicanor looked (and felt) for the 'dirt' disrupting flow to abdomens and lips; Elyn looked to RDT cassettes for proof of 'parasites' in bodies including my own; and Illaine, although unable to see agents of disease for herself, possessed the knowledge and authority to tell her patients where to go to have their illnesses unmasked. More importantly she, like all the other healers, had potent healing objects (drugs) at her disposal that could expel what was hidden inside. Along with *tari-tari*, incantations, visions, *rocorocco*, *silad*, *anting-anting*, healing oil, *sambong*, thermometers, RDTs, paracetamol, anti-malarials, cloth envelopes and coal, the very existence of disease was enacted alongside symbols of and constructs of authoritative professionalism (van der Geest & Whyte, 1989). As a result, the malaria or *malarya* that was defined and dealt with by professionals, although heterogeneous to some extent, hung together as a mutually intelligible sickness 'hidden' inside bodies that required qualified professionals with expert knowledge and tools to uncover or 'see' it in its acute phase when it manifested as *sakit* before being dealt with using specialised instruments. This contrasted with how patients, discussed in the next chapter, experienced these afflictions. Rather than be uncovered, seen and then extracted only by specialists, they needed to be dealt with through more mundane and everyday acts carried out in the long term that entailed keeping their entire bodies, social relations and even the cosmos in some sort of equilibrium in order to fulfil their strategic aim of 'feeling better' and retaining these feelings to stave off further affliction.

References

Bourdieu, P. (1977). *Outline of a theory of practice*. Cambridge University Press.

Brodwin, M. (1996). *Medicine and morality in Haiti: The contest for healing power*. Cambridge University Press.

Ewing, J. F. (1960). Birth customs of the Tawsug, compared with those of other Philippine groups. *Anthropological Quarterly, 33*(3).

Gesler, W. M. (1992). Therapeutic landscapes: Medical issues in light of the new cultural geography. *Social Science & Medicine, 34*(7), 735–746.

Hampshire, K. R., & Owusu, S. A. (2013). Grandfathers, Google, and dreams: Medical pluralism, globalization, and new healing encounters in Ghana. *Medical Anthropology: Cross-Cultural Studies in Health and Illness, 32*(3), 247–265.

Hampshire, K. R., Porter, G., Owusu, S. A., Tanle, A., & Abane, A. (2011). Out of the reach of children? Young people's health-seeking practices and agency in Africa's newly-emerging therapeutic landscapes. *Social Science & Medicine, 73*(5), 702–710.

Hörbst, V., & Wolf, A. (2014). ARVs and ARTs: Medicoscapes and the unequal place-making for biomedical treatments in sub-Saharan Africa. *Medical Anthropology Quarterly, 28*(2), 182–202.

Hsu, E. (2008). Medical pluralism. *Tobacco Control, 11*(1), 1–2.

Last, M. (1981). The importance of knowing about not knowing. *Social Science & Medicine, 15B*, 387–392.

Last, M., & Chavunduka, G. L. (Eds.). (1986). *The professionalisation of African medicine*. Manchester University Press in association with the International African Institute.

Leach, M. A., Fairhead, J. R., Millimouno, D., & Diallo, A. A. (2008). New therapeutic landscapes in Africa: Parental categories and practices in seeking infant health in the Republic of Guinea. *Social Science & Medicine, 66*(10), 2157–2167.

Macdonald, C. J.-H. (2007). *Uncultural behavior, an anthropological investigation of suicide in the southern Philippines*. University of Hawai'i Press.

Mallari, E., Lasco, G., Sayman, D. J., Amit, A. M. L., Balabanova, D., McKee, M., … Palafox, B. (2020). Connecting communities to primary care: A qualitative study on the roles, motivations and lived experiences of community health workers in the Philippines. *BMC Health Services Research, 20*(1), 860–860.

Marsland, R. (2007). The modern traditional healer: Locating "hybridity" in modern traditional medicine, Southern Tanzania. *Journal of Southern African Studies, 33*(4), 751–765.

Martin, D., Nettleton, S., Buse, C., Prior, L., & Twigg, J. (2015). Architecture and health care: A place for sociology. *Sociology of Health & Illness, 37*(7), 1007–1022.

Mendoza, R. L. (2009). is it really medicine? the traditional and alternative medicine act and informal health economy in the Philippines. *Asia-Pacific Journal of Public Health, 21*(3), 333–345.

Novellino, D. (2001). Pälawan attitudes towards illness. *Philippine Studies, 49*(1), 78–93.

Novellino, D. (2002). The relevance of myths and world views in Palawan classification, perceptions and management of Honey Bees. In J. R. Stepp, F. S. Wyndham, & R. K. Zarger (Eds.), *Ethnobiology and biocultural diversity: Proceedings of the 7th international congress of ethnobiology*. International Society of Ethnobiology.

O'Malley, J. (2004). Body as Teacher: The roles of clinical model and morphology in skill acquisition. In K. S. Oths & S. Z. Hinojosa (Eds.), *Healing by hand: Manual medicine and bonesetting in global perspective*. AltaMira Press.

Parkin, D. (1995). Latticed knowledge: Elimination and the dispersal of the unpalatable in Islam, medicine and anthropological theory. In R. Fardon (Ed.), *Counterwork: Managing knowledge in its diversity*. Routledge. London and New York.

Parkin, D. (2013). Medical crises and therapeutic talk. *Anthropology & Medicine, 20*(2), 124–141.

Revel, N. (1990). *Fleurs de Paroles Histoire Naturelle Pälawan (Vol. I, II, III)*. Editions Peeters.

Smyth, F. (2005). Medical geography: Therapeutic places, spaces and networks. *Progress in Human Geography, 29*(4), 488–495.

Tan, M. (2008). *Revisiting usog, pasma, kulam*. University of the Philippines Press.

Theriault, N. (2017). A forest of dreams: Ontological multiplicity and the fantasies of environmental government in the Philippines. *Political Geography, 58*, 114–127.

van der Geest, S., & Whyte, S. R. (1989). The charm of medicines: Metaphors and metonyms. *Medical Anthropology Quarterly, 3*(4), 345–367.

Wilson, K. (2003). Therapeutic landscapes and First Nations peoples: An exploration of culture, health and place. *Health & Place, 9*, 83–93.

6

Practices of Equilibrium

Introduction

So far in this book, I have described how various groups of people in Batraza have conceived of and practically dealt with a malaria (or *mala-rya*) that was largely experienced by others, namely members of the Pälawan community. In this chapter, I turn my attention to Pälawan people who actually suffered from a cluster of symptoms including fever, chills, headache, fatigue, stomach ache, body ache, vomiting and so on that they described as *malarya* or something very similar to it. When people experienced these ailments, their practices appeared united in that they were orientated towards gaining control over their bodies, social relations and the cosmos as a means with which to deal with both the acute and chronic nature of the *malarya* (Castillo-Carandang, 2009) and to fend off sickness and misfortune in the short and long terms. As was found across the Philippines, underlying many of these strategies was the principle of equilibrium (Tan, 2008) and the basic logic of prevention (through avoidance of imbalance) and then healing (through restoring balance). Among some I spoke to, this was achieved through *timbang* (Tagalog to weigh) and seemed to underscore much of social,

D. Iskander, *The Power of Parasites*, https://doi.org/10.1007/978-981-16-6764-0_6

environmental and cosmological life, which people described as existing in symbiotic relationship with the individual *bilug* (body). According to people I describe in this chapter, *malarya* 'came out' when equilibrium was disturbed, causing problems such as an inability to work, play, eat or socialise. Unlike the manifestations that could be isolated, 'seen' and treated within bodies in the acute stages of sickness by the professionals discussed in Chap. 5, the *malarya* described here by patients was enacted as an intra- and extra-bodily state and vulnerability and resistance to it was conceived of and built up over a lifetime. The practices that patients engaged in included attempts to weigh the body's interaction with the external environment or intrusive agents; efforts to maintain harmonious social relations and emotional lives; and endeavours to restore cosmological balance by appeasing or honouring relations between humans and the non-human world. I bring this to life through focussed descriptions of how a woman called Narcita dealt with her *malarya*, not through consulting professionals to uncover the unseen cause of her illness but through a combination of practical steps she and her family and friends took to restore her internal equilibrium, strengthen her *lama* (weak) body and increase her levels of *resistensiya* (Tagalog for resistance). As well as keeping the body in check, people worked towards keeping inter-personal relationships agreeable or 'cool'. This is exemplified by the situation of a lady named Isabelle. Due to distress in her family life, she described herself, and was labelled by others, as 'prone' to getting sick. Isabelle's main concern was not just to have her recurring and chronic fever and pain diagnosed or treated by one specific branch of healer in the short term but also to take active steps herself to mend the circumstances that led to her and her family's misfortune. Restoring equilibrium in relations in the long term entailed straddling different healing 'systems' in order to 'cool emotions'. The communal way in which sickness was dealt with among the Pälawan was no more evident than in the practice of *bayanihan*, whereby groups of people came together to help each other lift and relocate entire houses away from sites where *malarya* and fever came out due to the action of *diwata*. Bernas recounted how his father suffered from such an affliction and how the whole community shared the responsibility of restoring cosmological order on his behalf, an enterprise Bernas knew all too well in his role as *panglima* (leader) for his community.

When faced with sickness, people's practices appeared primarily motivated by their strategic concern to feel better and then also maintain these feelings of wellness in the future. Like healers, patients were less concerned with making sense of or even recreating ontological boundaries (e.g., between 'traditional' and 'biomedical' causes and treatments) in either labelling their conditions or taking particular steps to heal them. Rather, in order to bring an end to pain and subsequently ensure this state in the longer term, patients engaged in a sort of 'ethical choreography' (Stonington, 2020), consulting and interacting with a range of human and non-human actors, far beyond the health leaders, local government workers and professionals described thus far in this book in order to assemble 'good' ways to live.

Narcita's Weakened Body: Restoring Internal Equilibrium and Building Resistance

I sat and chatted to Tulima on her porch, a 14-year-old Pälawan girl who was taking part in the photovoice project that I was facilitating in her school. A middle-aged lady emerged from next door, wearing a brightly coloured *tadyong* (sarong) holding a bunch of leaves in her hand. 'This is *minan* (aunty) Narcita' Tulima told me. It transpired that Narcita had been preparing food for lunch in her house but knew Tulima was doing a project with me at the school to do with *malarya* so wanted to come and talk to me about her current situation. She handed me the bright green, long and aromatic leaves. 'Ah, this is *dangla* (*Vitex negundo L.*) or some people call it *lagundi* in Tagalog. You can easily tell because the leaves are in groups of five' Tulima told me as she splayed out her hand to mimic the arrangement of the foliage. I had come to speak to Tulima because in our photovoice sessions, in response to the question, 'What does malaria mean to you?' she had taken many pictures of various plants, herbal drinks, poultices and rubs and seemed very knowledgeable about health-related matters. However, she had also seemed a little reluctant to share her knowledge and had explained to me in private that she was shy about talking about *gamot* (Tagalog for medicines) in front of some of the others because she had inherited her knowledge from her *upuq* (grandparent, in this case grandfather)—a *mangagamot* (Tagalog for the one who heals). Although she enjoyed learning from him, she was conscious that some of the children in the class may laugh at her, particularly the few who were not Pälawan and therefore might not be familiar with these practices while those who were Pälawan may have admonished her for boasting about her knowledge. Nevertheless, she did want to share what she knew with me so a conversation out of the classroom was in order. '*Minan* Narcita has *sakit* (Tagalog for sickness/pain) for three days' Tulima went on and Narcita interjected, 'I picked these from my neighbour Mary-Jane down there on my way home. It is growing in the forest near her garden where she also grows *sambong* (*Blumea balsamifera* L.)—another good treatment for *malarya* but I already grow that myself.' She told me how from a young age, her father (Tulima's *upuq*) had shown her how to lightly pound the *dangla* leaves into a paste with a little warm water and then apply it to under the hottest parts of the body—the arms and legs—when someone was suffering with *egnew* (fever and chills). 'Immediately, the *linget* (sweat) will follow once you have applied the leaves and the *egnew* will subside. It depends on the person. With some people, *linget* will come immediately and the *egnew* will come out straight away. But with other people they have to put *dangla* many times. After two or three hours you repeat again until the *egnew* subsides completely.' I asked Narcita what she had done over the last three days to treat her *malarya* and she said 'nothing until now'. I then asked her if this was the first *gamot* she had used and she replied, 'No, I have taken one tablet of Paracetamol on the first day because I felt I did not want to eat or laugh and just wanted to lie down and rest. After I took it, I felt a little better so I rested more and did not take a bath before sleeping as I usually do. I did not want to make my body cold again. But the next day, I was still sick but had to go to the copra plantation because I had already made the arrangement with the owner to do *arawan* (Tagalog for wage labour).' She told me how her and her husband Ercito were employed as casual workers, earning around 200 PHS (£4) for every day that they worked on the plantation which was located down by the coast, quite far from their house, and that this was their main source of cash in addition to what she earned through selling some vegetables from their *uma* (swidden) field at a nearby *sari-sari* (road-side variety store). Ercito worked on the copra plantation far more that she did because the work was *meliut* (hard) involving retrieving and de-husking coconuts for many hours and constantly chopping wood to keep the kilns going. She occasionally worked there doing jobs such as weeding, planting or laying out the coconut flesh to dry in the sun or on the kiln if they needed some more money to help feed their three children or pay their school fees. Although she found *arawan* tiring, making her body ache with pain she said she liked the flexibility as if she had other work to do in the home or *uma*, particularly around planting and harvesting time, she did not register for *arawan*. However, she also pointed out that in instances such as this when she was sick, it was not possible to stay at home as she would lose the income and wanted to remain a good and trustworthy employee. She went on, 'I got *malarya* because I was out working in the heat doing *arawan*, laying the coconut shells in the sunshine to dry and got too hot but then it rained and the cold came inside my body'. I asked if you can get *malarya* any other way and she said she knew from health staff that you can also get *malarya* from *lamok* (Tagalog for mosquitoes) but said she wasn't aware of being bitten because she always slept under a mosquito net every night with her youngest children. While she acknowledged she could have been bitten at any time in the past because 'mosquitoes are all around', the reason she got sick this particular time was because of changes in climate which made her feel *lama* (weakened) causing the *malarya* in her body to 'come up'. She went on to tell me that she knew that her neighbour Mary-Jane had different plants near her house so she went to pick this one specifically [she didn't remember the name of it until Tulima reminded her] on the way home to make her lunch and that she would return to work again after she ate. She explained, 'I will keep drinking the juice from the leaves until I am better and will make sure to eat a lot of rice'. I ask her if she can go to see a professional or go to the *Barangay* Health Station to have a blood smear test as they are close by and she could get there and back in the time for lunch. She tells me that although they can give her stronger *gamot* (medicine), she can't go there because Ercito was still at work and her children at school so there was no-one from her close family to go with her. In any case, now that she has the *dangla*, she didn't feel it was urgent to go the health centre because she knew this would make her feel better. She tells me, '*dangla* and *sambong* are like a first-aid treatment for when you cannot get other kinds of stronger *gamot*. The main thing is not to take a bath and eat plenty of rice to stop the *malarya* coming up again in the future.'

Narcita's experience illustrates how sickness was conceived of and dealt with by many I met alongside wider notions of the body, health and well-being that were structured around equilibrium (Iskander, 2015) rather than more straightforward notions of cause and effect. Central to understanding why the *malarya* in Narcita's body 'came up' as result to changes in temperature and why remedy was sought in *dangla*, avoiding cold water, taking rest and eating rice was the principle of *timbang* (Tagalog to weigh). Multiple studies that explore health in various parts of the Philippines (Nichter & Nichter, 1996; Rosaldo, 1980) or amongst migrant Filipino groups (Anderson, 1983; Becker, 2003; Edman & Kameoka, 1997) have identified *timbang* to be at the heart of conceptions of health, social relationships and human interactions with their environment—illness therefore occurs as a result of disequilibrium when properties are not weighed against each other equally (Anderson, 1983). As Tan (2008) points out, 'equilibrium should not be interpreted in a narrow functionalist framework that emphasises maintenance of social equilibrium or the status quo. What is more important are the ways accumulation and excess are questioned, perceived as dangerous' (ibid., p. 138) and the notion of balance, rather than deflect individual responsibility, 'situates[s] the individual within a broader social framework where collective social responsibility is paramount' (ibid., p. 139).

The ideas behind prevention (the avoidance of inappropriate behaviours that caused disequilibrium) and cure (engaging in practices to restore equilibrium) were similar to principles found in other traditions in many contexts across the world based around humoral pathology. The extent to which, and the mechanisms through which, such ideas were transmitted to the Philippines from various external sources is contested (Anderson & Anderson, 1968; Hart, 1969; Orso, 1971; Rosaldo, 1971) but scholars tend to agree that conceptions found across the archipelago share features with many other traditions including Greek, Indian, Arabic or Chinese (ibid.). Among the Pälawan that I met, the notion of equilibrium was expressed as the relationship between the dichotomous attributes of *init* (hot) and *lamig* (cold) but also *basa* (wetness) and *pagkatuyo* (dryness) to a lesser extent which is unusual in many parts of the world where hot/cold complexes exist (Orso, 1971). People described how these were conferred in all living things by *Ampu* (ultimate creator or master) and were loosely associated with Tagalog concepts of *lupa* (earth/ground), *ulan* (rain), *araw* (sun) and *hangin* (wind) (Iskander, 2015). Remedies for illness were therefore conceived of in terms of appropriate actions, food, liquid, plants or medicines that also possessed and could counter these attributes (Rosaldo, 1971) to make people 'feel better', as Narcita emphasised.

As I have described elsewhere (Iskander, 2015), when talking to many Pälawan people, it became clear fairly quickly that many did not use a sole specific term for 'health' or 'healthy' instead articulating associated terms such as *masubug/kaya* (strong) or *metaba* (chubby) when discussing 'good health' as it were. Just like Narcita, people felt they were well or recovered from illness when they were able to work, socialise (often expressed as laughing/joking) or play and had a healthy appetite, describing the main indicator of ill-health as feeling *lama* or weakened (sometimes expressed as '*nanghihina ako*'—'I feel weak' in Tagalog) or vulnerable to fatigue (e.g., '*madaling mapagod ako*'—'I feel tired/exhausted easily' in Tagalog). As one lady put it, 'when the mosquito bites you, you will have *malarya* in your blood but you will not feel it if you are *masubug* but the moment you are *lama* then the *malarya* will wake up inside you'. Too much *sakit* was also an indicator of sickness and used in several Austronesian languages as synonymous with 'illness' (Tan, 2008, p. 21). In terms of malaria more specifically, the long history of official control and elimination efforts in Bataraza described throughout this book meant that it was something that everyone I met, adults and young people alike, knew about and mentioned when discussing health, often labelling a wide range of ailments under this umbrella term and describing their own illness as *malarya* regardless of any diagnosis from a professional. The vast majority of people I spoke to did not express exactly *what malarya* was beyond it being *sakit* and no reference was ever made to parasites among the Pälawan people I encountered. Causality wasn't directly expressed, with more expansive definitions being that *malarya* was disequilibrium inside the body, although never articulated in exactly those terms, and with no reference made to body 'humors'. Instead, people most often referred to internal bodily states and tended to use Tagalog terms to describe these: *malarya* was too much heat (*sobrang init*), too much cold (*sobrang lamig*), too much dryness (*sobrang pagkatuyo*), too much rain (*sobrang ulan*), too much dirt (*masyadong marumi*) inside the body and so on. In terms of the latter, as well as through the consumption of dirty food or water or coming into direct contact with dirt or rubbish, *lamok* (Tagalog for mosquitoes) were often cited as the main culprit for introducing, spreading or scattering dirt into the body through: biting people after having been in dirty places, entering the body directly through food or water or touching people's skin in water bodies used for swimming or washing (Iskander, 2015). Interestingly, disequilibrium was usually expressed as an excess rather than deficit of something. Similarly, the majority of people cited one or more manifestations of that state (what biomedicine refers to as symptoms), again using mostly Tagalog terms: *malarya was lagnat* (fever), *maginaw* (chills), *sakit ng ulo* (headache), *pagod* (fatigue), *hilo* (dizziness), *sakit sa tiyan* (stomach ache), *sakit ng katawan* (body ache) and *pagduduwal* (nausea), *nagsusuka* (vomiting) and so on.

Tulima was able to explain more about how internal bodily equilibrium was sometimes threatened and used some of her photographs to show me. Her thoughts were very much consistent with many of the themes that other children discussed in photovoice sessions. As described in Chap. 5, *pasma*, which loosely translated as 'exposure illness' (Frake, 1961), was cited by many adults and children as the reason for weakness in the body and *malarya* 'coming out'. As Tulima told me:

> [Pointing at image] In this picture you can see my mother under the tree being careful not to get too wet because rain with heat *(ulan-init* in Tagalog*)* is usually the cause of *malarya,* especially if you have been outside and then the rain comes suddenly or you take a cool bath or drink cold water or coconut juice then *pasma* and *malarya* will follow because your *resistensiya* is low at that time. Also, if you are taking exercise like jogging, basketball or playing with your friends then the body will become hot so you must make sure to rest and not expose your body to cold too fast to ensure everything is *timbang* so that it is the same. One more thing—too much work like doing *kaingin* or *arawan*, then over-fatigue. That's the reason. You have a lot of sweat and the sweat dries on your body making you cold and then you get *malarya* coming up for sure.

Her explanation of the sudden application of cold to hot was supported by the fact that so many people told me not to drink cool coconut water, especially in the morning (when temperatures were cooler) in order to prevent *malarya* and ensure my strength or *resistensiya*, defined as:

A popular health-related concept in the Philippines … [implying] a range of constructs including strength, absence of illness, ability to ward-off infections ("resistance" to infections), and being well enough to prevent serious illness. It could also describe a person's constitution like when a child is referred to as *malakas ang resistensya* ("having a strong resistance") which could mean he is not sickly, can easily fight off diseases (or some adverse condition), can bounce back to health more quickly, or is just generally strong and healthy. In contrast, someone with *"mahinang resistensya"* (weak resistance) would be more vulnerable to illness and take longer to recover from it. In the specific context of the Philippines, however, it also underscores individual responsibility and draws on concepts of social and political efficacy. (Acuin et al., 2009, p. 46)

These ideas also related to the equally common insistence that people must keep their bodily temperature in constant balance through a carefully selected and timed diet. Of paramount importance was to stay *busog* (Tagalog for fullness) and stave off *gutom* (Tagalog for hunger) by never missing a meal or *merienda* (Tagalog for snack). Mainly, though, it was through eating rice. Across the Philippines rice has long occupied an important place in both diet and culture (Aguilar, 2008) and lies at the very centre of Pälawan meals, social relations and spiritual life, as documented by many authors and mentioned briefly in Chap. 4 (Macdonald, 2007; Novellino, 2002; Smith, 2018, 2021). In terms of bodily health people reported the significance of rice mainly in terms of its warming qualities and ability to satiate like nothing else—a meal was not considered a meal unless it contained rice, and on its own rice was enough to be considered a meal precisely because no other food could fill one up in the same way. At times when rice was unobtainable or in short supply, which was relativity frequently (e.g., specific harvesting times, small yields or due to a lack of money), then substitutes such as cassava, taro and sweet potatoes were eaten in greater quantities but still seen as inferior to rice, and people often reported remaining hungry after their sole consumption. For the Pälawan, *adat pagbagi* (sharing) and *tabang* (mutual help) were crucial to the maintenance of convivial social relations as I go on to describe below. This and the overriding symbolic and cultural importance of rice were clearly manifested in the way swidden products were redistributed amongst family and community groups. As Macdonald (2007) explains:

> Within the local group (*rurungan*) the redistribution model is dominant, pooling at the centre and then redistributing resources. There is however, a major difference between the way the agricultural product (paddy, root crops, vegetables) is allocated between members of the group and the way game—and to a certain extent other wild products like honey or fishes—are redistributed in the same group. Essentially, swiddens were privately cultivated and their product privately owned by each household. However, I observed that sisters, who are the main agents in gathering these products, would tend to share their crops, visiting each other's fields together, gathering the products together, and partitioning them among themselves. In this way, through an exchange between siblings, the main dietary items, namely root crops and other vegetables, would circulate between household. Rice, on the other hand, the most prized item, was stored and not automatically redistributed but could be exchanged or sold. (Ibid., pp. 53–54)

Even outside the Pälawan community, the same principles seemed to apply. Sharing amongst family, neighbours and friends was extremely important but, again, there were certain limitations which my household constantly reminded me of when trying to educate me on the fundamentals of Filipino society. A common jesting turn of phrase I heard was that, if a hungry neighbour came to ask you for vegetables or money at any time of the day, then it was imperative to help them. However, if they asked you for rice in the evening, then you ought to refuse. The idea being that, due to the importance of rice, asking for it at night implied that the neighbour would not have time to return the favour by the end of the day and could therefore potentially incur an unpaid debt. The symbolic importance of the distribution of food was also reflected in the strong association between hunger and social exclusion including among my Pälawan participants. For example, in an early photovoice exercise, I asked the children to take a picture that reflected their mood. One boy named Aldwin took an image of the sky that he said revealed his feelings of loneliness that day as many of his friends were absent from school.

When I asked him how looking at the picture made him feel he replied '*nagugutom na ako*'—'I am getting hungry now'. Other children agreed—to be hungry was to be alone and *vice versa*. Crucially, lacking in either food or social relations could lower bodily *resistensiya* and lead to *malarya* 'coming out'.

The filling and warming qualities of rice were central to Narcita's insistence that the most important thing she could do to prevent the '*malarya* coming up again in the future' was to eat plenty of rice. Other foods too were described as being hot (e.g., legumes), cold (e.g., fruits), wet (e.g., okra) or dry (e.g., cassava), properties that similarly needed to be kept in check. In addition, some people highlighted the flavour profiles of salty, sweet, bitter and sour as also being important when considering what and when to eat as a means to keep the body strong against *malarya*. For example, in a focus group with 12 mothers from Tulima's school, in response to me asking how people get *malarya*, Mylene explained:

Inside [points to abdomen] we have a *baso-baso*—it is made of baso (Tagalog for glass) maybe. … When we eat food that is *maasim* (sour) like green mango or vinegar it will go to the *baso-baso* and stir up the *malarya* there and it will run to the whole body. If it is not treated then it can get to a higher degree and become *falciparum*. … When we were young our parents told us not to eat mango or food that is *maasim* especially when it is hot, because it will affect the *baso-baso* and we noticed when we were sick our parents would give us Camoquin (Amodiaquine) or Aralen (Chloroquine) then more recently Chloroquine when we were sick.

The notion that *malarya* was somehow always present in the body, even to a low degree, but had the potential to build up over a lifetime was expressed by most people that I spoke to who felt it was rather unproblematic on the whole at such low levels but increased at particularly vulnerable times in life when the body was weak. As the women go on to discuss:

Nelsa: When you are born as a Filipino, *malarya* it is there already inside your body.
Rosely: Yes, I agree that when we are born, we have that *malarya* inside … because even young babies experience fever and chills. But the *malarya* in the past when we were babies was absolutely stronger than in the

present day because right now there are a lot of midwives and BHWs organised by the government and they are distributing mosquito nets and doing programmes so now it is so much less strong.

Melita: I think the reason sometimes you are sick and sometimes not sick is because you eat food that is against whatever sickness is in your *baso-baso* and it makes you weak but if you eat food that is not against it then you will be OK. It is not forbidden to eat mango or vinegar but just not too much—you must ensure you have just a little now and then. Also, coconut juice or sugar cane, it is the same because they are also *matamis* (sweet) and *maasim* (sour). Our parents could always tell is we had *malarya* because they could feel the *baso-baso* like that sticking out on the outside

Me: Is there anything else that would make a person get *malarya*?

Rosely: Maybe from mosquito bites bringing too much dirt that also makes your body weak.

When malaria was confirmed at the Rural Health Clinic, staff like Danny and Maria whom I discussed in Chap. 3 would inform patients whether their case was mild or severe. As most malaria infections in Bataraza were due to *Plasmodium falciparum*, this was expressed as '*falciparum* 1 or *falciparum* 2' to indicate the severity. Many people said that this confirmed that *malarya* was always in the body but could be *tumaas* (Tagalog for increased, topped up) throughout one's life. A young man named Dormin had suffered multiple attacks of *malarya* as a young boy and explained:

I am careful now to always stay strong and eat plenty of vegetables and rice. Maybe I did not take enough care for that when I was young. I don't know, but maybe, just maybe, you get bitten by a mosquito so it adds to your *malarya* already in your body. Why else would it increase? Before, maybe you just have *malarya*, then later you have *falciparum* 3 some years later. How is that possible? I think even if you are being treated with Chloroquine or Primaquine, it's not 100% that the *malarya* is never taken away from your body so it must always remain there a little and that is how I got it so many times in my life—through not taking enough care or maybe from doing bad things and not being *mehubrej* (a good person). So, it's still stuck in there!

Participants therefore distinguished between the intensity of sicknesses but did not make any reference to different kinds of malaria in the way that health staff did. Very few participants referred to other species such as *'vixax'* and none to *'malariae'*, although there were infections with these two species in Bataraza. Some studies of malaria in other parts of the Philippines found that participants categorised different sorts of malaria such as that of the liver (*malarya sa atay*), blood (*dugo*) or stomach (*pali*) (Miguel et al., 1998). In the area of Morong, people recognised up to 20 different types (Espino et al., 1997) of the disease. I did not find this, instead only that people associated the strongest level of *malarya—falciparum 4*—with the brain. Danny had told me that since he had been in office (since 2004), there were very few cases of cerebral malaria—the most severe neurological complication of infection with *Plasmodium falciparum*. However, people reported that they had seen or heard of members of their community who had suffered long-term effects of *malarya* in the 'head' that had affected their mental state. By the time levels had reached *falciparum 4*, *malarya* was thought to be able to *paglalakbay* (Tagalog for travel) or *tumakbo* (Tagalog for run) to the highest part of the body. As Sita told me:

> *Falciparum* is the same as *malarya* but it is a higher degree of sickness because it is too much, it runs to the brain and sometimes you are bed ridden. The most severe is *falciparum* 4. If you get that then you can become crazy. In Bataraza there a lot of crazy people from *malarya*. That is why *malarya* can be very dangerous if you do not keep your body strong from attack.

As well as keeping individual bodies in balance, many people spoke of the importance of keeping familial and social relations in similar check; otherwise groups of people were also vulnerable to weakness, making resistance even harder to build up as demonstrated by Isabelle's situation.

Isabelle's Chronic Fever: The 'second spear', Fatalism and Straddling Different Systems to Cool Emotions

While Ramil and I were conducting interviews with adult caregivers at the school to assess the impact of photovoice on children, their families and the wider community, one student's mother, who I call Isabelle, apologised for not attending her scheduled time slot with me the previous week and explained that she had had another attack of her recurring sickness—fever, chills, headaches and body ache, so severe that she had had to take to her bed for four or five days. I took the opportunity to ask her more about her condition and she recounted how it had started many years ago:

> I was up there [pointing towards the forest] doing *kaingin* and harvesting the bananas and suddenly I felt something hit me from the back and then there was *sakit* (pain) all the way in my body. Some months later, my eldest daughter came home from Puerto and she asked me if she could have some bananas to take back with her to college. I told her to go up there and get them from our *kaingin* field but she said no and we argued and my husband told me to go there and collect them for her. When I was there, I also collected some corn and was carrying it home in a large basket on my back. When I was walking on the road, I felt someone was pulling my basket and I felt a sharp pain again in my back as if someone had pushed me. I looked around to see who had pushed me and there was no one there so I was shouting for them to stop but then I knew then it was *bati* because there was no person there. I ran home and from that time on I have had pain in my neck and shoulders and back. Since then, maybe years ago now, I get sick all the time with this pain and fever. I went to the RHU (Rural Health Unit) for treatment but they told me 'this is not *malarya* even though it looks the same so we cannot treat it'. I went to the *albularyo* (Tagalog for herbalist) and he gave me *gamot* but still I keep getting sick again and again. I can prove it is related to *bati* because I get it when I go up there to the *kaingin* and then I go to the *albularyo* and I feel better for a short time but then I go there again sometime later to get the bananas or corn and I feel something attack me and then I get sick again. Some people are *madaling kapitan ng sakit* (prone to getting sick in Tagalog) more than others and I am prone. It means you have had difficulties in your life or done bad things that have *bagabagin* (Tagalog for brought distress) and maybe it will affect not just you but even your relations in the future. Maybe that day it was because I had argued with my daughter and husband and we had not been *meingasiq* (loving, compassionate, generous). Sometimes it is because your *kagurangurangan* (ancestors) hurt the *diwata* when they were still alive in the past and so now the *diwata* continue to attack you or sometimes you could have touched or hurt the *diwata* directly in this life without knowing

and so you are prone to *bati*. It is bad to be prone. But you can make peace with your family and even the *kagurangurangan* or *diwata* by making *atang* (offerings of food in Tagalog) to them. At the moment, my family is discussing together whether or not I should make the *atang* again. I already did it some time ago but maybe it was not enough. It is a big decision because you have to go to see the *albularyo* and maybe he will ask you for rice and even a chicken or some cigarettes so we are discussing now with the family if I should do it [or not]. I want to do it as maybe it will help to cool the liver (meaning to cool emotions) and make me feel better.

Following the interview, Ramil engaged in a long discussion with Isabelle as I carried on with another interview. However, as they parted, I noted that she ended the conversation with a long sigh and shrug uttering a phrase I had heard a lot, '*bahala-na*', which Ramil translated as 'whatever happens happens'. I asked Ramil what she meant and he replied, 'this is a complex case, maybe she means she is resigned to her fate'. Once Isabelle had left, Ramil provided his own explanation for Isabelle's illness:

This is a very sad situation and you know, her illness is because of her life situation. Lately, her 14-year-old daughter was hurt by a man who is close with a local politician. Although he admitted it, his wife is defending him in public. I was involved in the case to have the girl removed to Peurto for her own protection and since then the family have not seen her and their relations with the politician are heated. Isabelle has been to Puerto twice to try to find her daughter but cannot get any information about where she is exactly. She says she will go again to Puerto next week and wanted my help to try and find her. This is what contributes to being prone as she says. Like how do you say in English, her 'misfortune in life' or her 'emotional distress'. This is a very sad situation for their family—in fact she has had so many problems in the past and now this misfortune is spreading to her daughter. They are trying to resolve things with the politician's people so maybe when these issues are dealt with, they will have peace. You know, every Filipino will tell you that, whatever their religion is, it is not just in the body, but mind and even in the soul that needs to be in balance. In fact, we all must be at peace with each other in order to be strong, to build up resistance to misfortune.

Isabelle's plight was indicative of how for many, their 'life situation' as Ramil described it, was intimately linked to their sense of vulnerability to illness and ability to build resistance. There appeared to be a distinct temporal, spatial, social and—crucially—ethical quality to both. This was hinted at earlier in Dormin's sense of his past carelessness over his body or 'bad' acts that had increased his susceptibility to repeated bouts of *malarya* and Isabelle's concern that her accumulated 'distress' from 'difficulties' and 'bad' deeds would have repercussions not just for herself but for her whole family in the future, unless remedied. Vulnerability to *bati* was talked about by most people and one man, Seylin, explained to me that 'no one can avoid *bati*. But if you are prone to it then you will experience it wherever you go and be in many places. There are some people that are attractive to the *diwata* in the mountain or forest and other people that are not attractive but it is a little sensitive to discuss these matters because it means something bad to be prone'. The lack of linearity surrounding illness echoed Evans-Pritchard's (1937) description of the practices he observed among the Azande of North Central Africa which led him to argue that witchcraft acted as 'second spear' or *umbaga*, explaining *why* certain events were harmful to humans but not necessarily *how* they came to happen when they did. For example, when a man was killed by an elephant, the first spear or acute cause was the elephant but the second more chronic cause was witchcraft, leading the universe to place the victim in that particular situation at that particular time. Both spears were necessary to harm (ibid.). Isabelle's second spear was her 'misfortune' in life and 'emotional distress', built up over a lifetime, involving many actors ranging from the politician's contact to her dead ancestors. This explained why she was attacked in her swidden field at the time she was. Both the first and second spears were necessary for her illness to take place and in this way pointed to both the acute and the chronic nature (Castillo-Carandang, 2009) of *malarya* and *bati* (which presented as very similar). While the professionals described in Chap. 5 dealt with sickness in its acute phase within the body, people such as Narcita and Isabelle worked to reconcile past, present and future relations both within and external to their own bodies.

Although Ramil conjectured that Isabelle's expression of '*bahala-na*' may have suggested that she was 'resigned to her fate', little about her account indicated that she was not motivated to engage in action to try and improve her situation and change the course of events for herself and her family. Her intentional practices ranged from repeatedly taking *gamot* prescribed by the *albularyo*, going to Puerto to find her daughter and making *atang* to the *diwata* as a means to cool emotions (which I discuss further below). Rather than simply imply a world-view of fatalism (Gripaldo, 2005), the expression which was commonly used across the Philippines was more ambiguous. Gripaldo (2005) offered six meanings, some of which are come/happen what may; do what you want, it's up to you, but be ready for the consequences; and let it be. *Bahala-na* and fatalism have thus been cited as 'barriers' to prompt health-seeking behaviour amongst various Filipino groups in arenas such as breast cancer (Wong-Kim, 2007) and other life-threatening situations (McLaughlin & Braun, 1998; Vance, 1995). I found that some healthcare professionals I met also expressed this sentiment. For example, a doctor in a private hospital explained to me how the 'resignation' that he saw in his Pälawan patients had fatal consequences:

> I have learnt to be very careful about telling patients if they were seriously ill as they immediately want to kill themselves. If someone is told they had fatal illness they would go home straight away and will not want to stay in the hospital even if we think there is something we can do to help them or to relieve the pain.

However, consistent with Tan's (2013) recent review of the concept, I found that the *bahala-na* 'attitude', as it were, did not exclude prompt action nor an individual sense of responsibility. Tan cites a reinterpretation of *bahala-na* by Lagmay (1993) who observed that:

> The person who says "*bahala na*" does not avoid a problem; instead, he or she remains committed to meeting the problem, even while recognizing the difficulties or seriousness of it. Important for Lagmay was the improvisation or extemporization, as the person looks for ways to solve the problem. (Tan, 2013)

When discussing the death of a close family member, one friend used the phrase and immediately followed it with 'we Filipinos know that we must enjoy life because one day you are here and the next not—there is nothing to stop it'. As Tan (2013) suggests, when faced with the uncertainly inherent in illness, the concept of *bahala-na* perhaps 'emboldened' rather than discouraged action as people resigned themselves not to a predetermined fate, but to the idea that 'I'm going to do what I can' in this situation as one must live from one moment to the next (ibid.).

Finally, in terms of what it is that people such as Isabelle did in the face of such complex misfortune, practices were not confined within one medical 'system' as they were orientated around principals of ethics and doing 'good'. Patients, just like the professionals I described in Chap. 5, also seemed to 'straddle', transcend and contest (Hampshire & Owusu, 2013; Marsland, 2007; McMillen, 2004) different therapeutic traditions, blurring the boundaries between various 'systems' of knowledge and practice. Narcita took paracetamol and *dangla* and Isabelle consulted healers from different backgrounds. Like many I encountered, they did not even make clear divisions between 'biomedical' and 'folk'; 'modern' and 'traditional'; 'formal' and 'informal' forms of care. In fact, during discussions, most people did not really understand why I asked questions that implied any distinction at all between 'herbal' and 'non-herbal' medicines as the word *gamot* applied to all. Similarly, as Tulima articulated when describing her grandfather, the word *mangagamot* was used to describe all kinds of healers ranging from *balyans* and *manghihilots* to midwives and doctors in the health clinic with distinctions being rather arbitrary, to some extent. This straddling of systems was significant because the vast majority of health-related literature centres around the idea of 'first resort' documenting what people initially do in response to an illness episode. Implicit is the idea that there are objective, demarcated, health-specific 'behaviours' that can be separated out from the situated context in which they emerge and that there is an element of linearity and predictability to such behaviours. I even fell into this trap, asking Narcita what was the 'first' thing she had done to treat her *malarya*. As a result, some 'practices' are brought to the foreground such as taking medicines or consulting professionals while other wider, situated, non-linear practices are ignored such as Narcita's resting and avoidance of taking a cool bath. In addition, her course of action was clearly not just 'simply a function of knowledge or beliefs' (Jones & Williams, 2004, p. 157) as it was entirely contingent on the 'here and now'. The convenient location and generosity of her neighbour Mary-Jane meant she was able to procure some *dangla* from her garden on the way home while the absence of her husband and children meant she could not go to the health clinic. Her commitment to work and compulsion to keep the good favour of her employer impeded her ability to do more but the teachings of her deceased father meant she had 'first-aid' treatments at her immediate disposal. Health and social realities were so intimately woven together that it was impossible, if not meaningless, to try to isolate and identify specific health 'behaviours' and recreate the order in which they occurred, divorced of their incorporation in the 'social, affective, material and interrelational features of human activity' (Cohn, 2014, p. 159).

As for Isabelle, the messiness of her chronic fever was very much tied to the emotional life of her and her family and therefore took on an even more pronounced ethical dimension. She expressed quite directly that the lack of being *meingasiq* (loving, compassionate, generous) with her immediate family may have sparked the first attack of *diwata* and that now her practices were orientated around 'cooling the liver'. For the Pälawan, the *atej* or liver was the seat of emotions, memory and sensitivity— of morality in other words (Macdonald, 2007). To be 'good-livered' expressed a similar sentiment to being good-hearted in English and suggested that the cooling of the liver that Isabelle strove for was not only a strategy to fend off the rising body heat associated with febrile illness but also her feelings of anger, shame and distress in favour of compassion, love and generosity, which for many were the main constituents of a sense of moral worth (Macdonald, 2007). Efforts she made to appease the angered *diwata* such as *atang* and improving relations with the local politician and his allies were key to Isabelle's attempts at being *mehubrej* (a good person) as Dormin put it. As the next example shows, this ethical endeavour was a collective as much as a personal one and sometimes required the help of the whole community.

Moving the House of Bernas' Father: Communal Attempts to Balance the Cosmos

A common sight in Pälawan villages was that of the remnants of old *bena* (houses): stilt foundations holding nothing above them, a single rotting post or discarded roofing materials. While some were no doubt abandoned due to wear and tear, destruction from the elements or simply a relocation due to economic or social reasons, an additional practice amongst the Pälawan was also *bayanihan*—the purposeful lifting and moving of whole houses following an illness. I witnessed this practice when I was invited to join a celebration in an upland community consisting of around 30 households under the jurisdiction of *panglima* Vidly. The family that owned the house had gone to significant lengths to mark this occasion. A pig had been slaughtered and speakers, which were blaring out pop music when I arrived, had been hired from the town to add to the festive ambiance. The reason for this large gathering was that the group had come together to carry the family's house only 20 metres or so further along the track because the mother had been sick—with what Vidly told me was her second attack of *malarya* in as many months—had been advised by an *albularyo* that this was the best course of action to take. Over lunch, I asked one of the attendees whom I had come to know well, *panglima* Bernas, about this practice, which he said had been part of Pälawan culture from 'time immemorial'. He recounted his own experience when his father had been struck by a similar illness many years before:

If a person has a problem, his problem is not only his own problem but we consider it a shared problem of the whole community and everyone must help in that to help the person to feel better. That is very important in our culture to make everyone have a good life here. If it's a sickness like sweating and fever then, for sure, the cause of the sickness is the location of the house especially if the sweat is a lot and they have a high temperature and chills. This is particularly if the sweating and chills is repeating like one time in the morning and then again in the afternoon then, absolutely, the cause is because of the location of the house. Inside the ground we cannot see what it is—maybe bad *diwata*. For example, my father, built a very nice house with a very nice nipa roof and big *legwas* (yard) for growing many vegetables. It was a very big house with two big rooms and space for many of us to sleep. After three months he became very sick. He was sweating in the morning and then again in the afternoon. So, he called his younger brother who knew about these things and said 'please come and do the *tari-tari* (diagnostic procedure) in my house because I am feeling sick in the morning and the afternoon'. So, he came and told my father to leave the house for a few minutes. He then started talking to someone in the house but it wasn't a person that you could see so maybe it was some *diwata*. When my father was going up the ladder of his neighbour's house, he suddenly felt that the sickness had gone. When he left his own house, he was immediately better so his brother said that we must wait a little more until the afternoon and see what would happen next. My father stayed with the neighbour and had some food together with him. By the afternoon, my father got well and so it confirmed that it was the house for sure. He stayed in the neighbour's house one more night and then the next day decided to move our house from that area where he built it—maybe he had disturbed the *diwata* who owned that place. So, we got all the families together— maybe about 30 families and moved the house just a little way. It was such a big house that it was a hard job because so many pieces of bamboo had to tied together to make a big frame and maybe 20 men carried the house resting that bamboo on their shoulders with the house above. Everyone helped in that. Once he moved the house, he did not get any more sicknesses like that related to the location of the house. That's why *bayanihan* is a culture passed down from our *kagurangurangan*; it's not from Muslims or anything—just from *our* culture.

Bernas was clear that practices orientated around *adat pagbagi* (sharing) and *tabang* (mutual help) were central to both *bayanihan* and Pälawan culture more generally. As well as pointing to the communal way in which *malarya* and fever were dealt with among people I met, this case, like Isabelle's, also illustrated the way in which non-humans who enlivened the landscape were very much implicated in this interrelational way of being. Hirsch and O'Hanlon (1995) articulate how landscapes become constructed though people's attempts to realise what is in the background (sites of potentiality) within 'foreground landscapes' (ibid., pp. 3–5), becoming part of people as much as people become part of them (Ingold, 1993, p. 154). Avoiding, assuaging and appeasing figures in the 'background' such as *Ampu*, *diwata* and a whole host of other non-human actors was part of everyday life for most people. A day didn't go by when I wasn't told to rather light-heartedly to stay away from 'that big tree over there where the angry *diwata* lives' or walk round 'that mound that is the dwarf's home' in order to avoid getting sick. Children in particular were especially adept at traversing the landscape together and I often saw them holding hands or clumping together in groups to safely run past potentially dangerous places. These sorts of mundane practices were woven into the fabric of everyday life and went unnoticed for the most part to the point that people appeared 'embodied in place and emplaced in body' (Langton, 2002, p. 260). Even after a few weeks of being in Bataraza, I myself began to see them as rather unremarkable and quotidian acts, very much incorporating them into my ways of being in the place. However, when affliction did arise, as has been made clear in this chapter, more exceptional action was taken in the form of the *atang* such as those made by Isabelle, *bayanihan* conducted by Bernas' father or even, in the past at least, the sacrifice of human life. As *panglima*, one of Bernas' main duties was to deal with infringements of *adat* (customary law) that threatened the moral order, angered unseen actors inhabiting the landscape and resulted in sicknesses of several kinds. As he explains:

> Sometimes there is crime committed here like if a boy steals a coconut or there is fighting between couples or adultery but these are human problems and we can solve that if we talk together with the people. The most serious offence is *sumbang* (incest), for example between first cousins or the worst kind is between grandparents. If that happens then there will be a curse for the whole community from the *tandayag* (a large fish-like monster said to reside in the ocean). When *sumbang* happens, the *tandayag* will be angry and go to the mountains and make too much sunlight or extreme heat for so many days. *Ampu* will send the rain to cool the mountain resulting in too much rain, sometimes for many months. If that happens, it is very bad for our *kaingin* and could mean the harvest is weak. In my father's time the punishment for *sumbang* was to kill the couple either by tying them up at the top of the mountain exposing them to the heat to make the rain come or by putting them in a basket with heavy rocks and throwing them into the ocean so that the heat comes. Now, we are not allowed to do this anymore because the government forbade it so if *sumbang* happens we must

hold a meeting as *panglima* with the whole tribal council and decide on the penalty. Nowadays, a small cut will be made at the top of the thigh—usually only of the man—to draw a little blood which is put on a plate and the plate is thrown into the ocean. If the waves become bigger then it means the *tandayag* has accepted that offer of peace and the heat or rain will go and maybe the harvest will be saved. Other times, the couple may have to pay a very large fine of 10,000 pesos. It happened just three months ago in one area and the *panglima* there performed the cutting of the boy near the river because he was found to have relations with his niece. They had to give 350 plates as their penalty which were distributed to everyone in the *barangay* for them to use in their *kaingin*. Before you sew the rice in the *kaingin*, it is very important to do the *pinadungan* and make a platform or small house with a nice floor in the middle of the *kaingin*. On a plate you must put seven seeds of rice and leave it there in that little house overnight and pray for no bad effects from *sambung*. In the morning, when you come back, if everything is in its place and no seeds are lost then you know the harvest will be good this year and there will not be too much heat or too much rain. But, when the rice starts to grow, you must watch to see if the leaves are stunted because if that happened then you know there has been *sambung* somewhere and maybe the *panglima* in that area did not arrange any penalty or plates and the *tandayag* is still angry. That has happened here, many times now, there is too much heat or rainy days. The rain does not always come on time so we know then that *sumbang* has happened and we try to call all the *panglimas* together to make sure they punish it. But maybe since we are not allowed to kill the people who did that *sumbang*, it is not enough—I don't know. If we do not have rice then the whole community is affected. If we are hungry then our bodies will be *lama* (weakened) and we will be sick or even die. That's why the part of the *panglima* is so important for the whole community so that through him they can keep the climate in balance and avoid the curse for everyone from bad actions like *sambung*.

Conclusion

Bernas' final words reinforce just how interlinked the individual body, the social body and the cosmological body were for the people I described in this chapter. In order to prevent weakness, build resistance and feel better in the face of illness, people such as Narcita, Isabelle and Bernas worked to balance different elements including their bodies, emotions and relations with human and non-human entities as a means to deal with the acute and chronic nature of *malarya* (Castillo-Carandang, 2009), which itself 'came out' as a result of a complex web of imbalanced circumstances and relations. This orientation towards feeling better also had a moral quality as all expressed a desire to do 'good' in some way, whether it was to regain the individual bodily strength needed to eat, work and socialise in the case of Narcita, cool the hot emotions in social relations causing so much distress in the case of Isabelle and her family or swiftly deal with incest that had the potential to bring on a poor harvest and sickness to the entire community in the case of Bernas. Following Stonington (2020), I suggest that these actors were engaged in a kind of 'ethical choreography', both strategising and improvising in practical, bodily ways to assemble the right elements needed to do good in life. In this everyday ethical space, the *malarya* that was enacted as an intra- and extra-bodily state appeared to be co-opted into (un)conscious strategies of maintaining equilibrium on the part of people who dealt with a different kind of *malarya* to the ones handled by health leaders, local government actors and professionals described thus far in this book. In the final chapter that follows I reflect on this multi-faceted nature of disease and offer my thoughts on what the people of Bataraza showed me about the power of malaria parasites.

References

Acuin, C. S., Vargas, A. S., & Cordero, C. P. (2009). Formative research to develop and test messages to educate mothers on Zinc supplementation in childhood Diarrhea. *Acta Medica Philippina, 43*(4), 43–51.

Aguilar, F. V. J. (2008). *Rice in the Filipino diet and culture*. Philippine Institute for Development Studies.

Anderson, E. N., & Anderson, M. L. (1968). Folk medicine in rural Hong Kong. *Etnoiatria, 2*(1), 22–28.

Anderson, J. N. (1983). Health and illness in Pilipino immigrants. *Western Journal of Medicine, 139*, 811–819.

Becker, G. (2003). Cultural expressions of bodily awareness among chronically Ill Filipino Americans. *Annals of Family Medicine, 1*(2), 113–118.

Castillo-Carandang, N. T. (2009). Notions of risk and vulnerability to malaria. *Acta Medica Philippina, 43*(3), 48–55.

Cohn, S. (2014). From health behaviours to health practices: An introduction. *Sociology of Health & Illness, 36*(2), 57–162.

Edman, J. L., & Kameoka, V. A. (1997). Cultural differences in illness schemas: An analysis of Filipino and American illness attributions. *Journal of Cross-Cultural Psychology, 28*(3), 252–265.

Espino, F., Manderson, L., Acuin, C., Domingo, F., & Ventura, E. (1997). Perceptions of malaria in a low endemic area in the Philippines: Transmission and prevention of disease. *Acta Tropica, 63*(4), 221–239.

Evans-Pritchard, E. E. (1937). *Witchcraft, oracles and magic among the Azande.* Oxford University Press.

Frake, C. O. (1961). The diagnosis of disease among the Subanun of Mindanao. *American Anthropologist, 63*(1), 113–132.

Gripaldo, R. M. (2005). Bahala na: A philosophical analysis. In R. M. Gripaldo (Ed.), *Filipino cultural traits* (pp. 203–220). Claro R. Ceniza Lectures: Council for Research in Values and Philosophy.

Hampshire, K. R., & Owusu, S. A. (2013). Grandfathers, Google, and dreams: Medical pluralism, globalization, and new healing encounters in Ghana. *Medical Anthropology: Cross-Cultural Studies in Health and Illness, 32*(3), 247–265.

Hart, D. V. (1969). *Bisayan Filipino and Malayan humoral pathologies: Folk medicine and ethnohistory in Southeast Asia.* Southeast Asia Program, Cornell University.

Hirsch, E., & O'Hanlon, M. (Eds.). (1995). *The anthropology of landscape: Perspectives on place and space.* Vol. Oxford Studies in Social and Cultural Anthropology. Clarendon Press.

Ingold, T. (1993). The temporality of the landscape. *World Archaeology, 25*(2), 152–174.

Iskander, D. (2015). Re-imaging malaria in the Philippines: How photovoice can help to re-imagine malaria. *Malaria Journal, 14*(1), 257.

Jones, C. O., & Williams, H. A. (2004). The social burden of malaria: What are we measuring? *The American Journal of Tropical Medicine and Hygien, 71*(2 Suppl), 156–161.

Lagmay, A. V. (1993). Bahala na! *Philippine Journal of Psychology, 26*(26), 31–36.

Langton, M. (2002). The edge of the sacred, the edge of death: Sensual inscriptions. In B. David & M. Wilson (Eds.), *Inscribed landscapes: Marking and making place* (pp. 253–269). University Of Hawai'i Press.

Macdonald, C. J.-H. (2007). *Uncultural behavior, an anthropological investigation of suicide in the southern Philippines.* University of Hawai'i Press.

Marsland, R. (2007). The modern traditional healer: Locating "hybridity" in modern traditional medicine, Southern Tanzania. *Journal of Southern African Studies, 33*(4), 751–765.

McLaughlin, L. A., & Braun, K. L. (1998). Asian and Pacific Islander cultural values: Considerations for health care decision making. *Health & Social Work, 23*(2), 116–126.

McMillen, H. (2004). The adapting healer: Pioneering through shifting epidemiological and sociocultural landscapes. *Social Science & Medicine, 59*(5), 889–902.

Miguel, C. A., Manderson, L., & Lansang, M. A. (1998). Patterns of treatment for malaria in Tayabas, The Philippines: implications for control. *Tropical Medicine & International Health, 3*(5), 413–421.

Nichter, M., & Nichter, M. (1996). Acute respiratory illness: Popular health culture and mothers knowledge in the Philippines. In M. Nichter & M. Nichter (Eds.), *Anthropology and international health: Asian case studies* (2nd ed.). Gordon & Breach.

Novellino, D. (2002). The relevance of myths and world views in palawan classification, perceptions and management of Honey Bees. In J. R. Stepp, F. S. Wyndham, & R. K. Zarger (Eds.), *Ethnobiology and biocultural diversity: Proceedings of the 7th international congress of ethnobiology.* International Society of Ethnobiology.

Orso, E. (1971). Review of Bisayan Filipino and Malayan humoral pathologies: Folk medicine and ethnohistory in Southeast Asia. Data Paper: No. 76. *American Anthropologist, 73*(2), 399–400.

Rosaldo, M. Z. (1980). *Knowledge and passion: Ilongot notions of self and social life.* Cambridge University Press.

Rosaldo, R. (1971). Review of Bisayan Filipino and Malayan humoral pathologies: Folk medicine and ethnohistory in Southeast Asia. Data Paper: No. 76. *Bijdragen tot de Taal-, Land- en Volkenkunde, 127*, 403–406.

Smith, W. (2018). Weather from incest: The politics of indigenous climate change knowledge on Palawan Island, the Philippines. *The Australian Journal of Anthropology, 29*(3), 265–281.

Smith, W. (2021). *Mountains of blame climate and culpability in the Philippine Uplands / Will Smith.* Seattle University of Washington Press.

Stonington, S. D. (2020). Karma masters: The ethical wound, hauntological choreography, and complex personhood in Thailand. *American Anthropologist, 122*(4), 759–770.

Tan, M. (2008). *Revisiting usog, pasma, kulam.* University of the Philippines Press.

Tan, M. (2013). Bahala na. *Philippine Daily Inquirer.*

Vance, A. R. (1995). Filipino Americans. In J. N. Giger & R. E. Davidhizar (Eds.), *Transcultural nursing: Assessment and intervention* (2nd ed., pp. 279–401). Mosby Year Book.

Wong-Kim, E. C. (2007). Promoting health among Asian American Population groups by using key informants: A case study. In M. V. Kline & R. M. Huff (Eds.), *Health promotion in multicultural populations: A handbook for practitioners and students.* Sage.

7

Conclusion

Early in 2014, I went to visit Danny at his house. While I'd been back home in the United Kingdom, celebrating Christmas with my family, he had been in hospital, seriously ill with pneumonia. Although he'd been discharged some weeks before, I found him weak, gaunt and in obvious discomfort. Danny being Danny, however, still had the RHU, his staff and his patients at the forefront of his mind. As we sat on his porch, he laboured through difficult breaths to tell me his 'malaria news'. He had heard that it was likely that the Global Fund would renew their grant allocation for Palawan so he was feeling positive that he and his team would be able to reach the target of 'a malaria-free' Bataraza in the coming years. He joked that if I ever returned to do more fieldwork, I would have to find a new topic. As he sipped some water through a straw, he looked over at the children playing basketball in his yard and said, 'malaria is just like that ball. While it is with us, we must keep juggling it, passing it around, until one day, because of everyone's effort, it might be thrown so high into the sky it will never come back.' Danny and the people I have described in this book showed me exactly this: that in Bataraza, malaria was indeed at the centre of a sort of 'game' (Bourdieu, 1977) that

© The Author(s), under exclusive license to Springer Nature Singapore Pte Ltd. 2021 **197**
D. Iskander, *The Power of Parasites*, https://doi.org/10.1007/978-981-16-6764-0_7

they, and me, were all tangled up in. And just like the ball, malaria was very much in our hands.

However, rather than be at the centre of just one game, it was entangled within many games, each with its own set of rules. On top of that, more than one ball was passed between more than one team, including past Spanish, American and Japanese colonisers; contemporary health leaders such as Danny, Renya and Michael; government officials like the Mayor, *Barangay* Captains and Pälawan Chieftains; professionals such as Sario, Nicanor, Elyn and Illaine; members of the Pälawan community including Narcita, Isabelle and *panglima* Bernas; and now, too, an anthropologist with her notebooks. Our court was made up Bourdieu's (1977) overlapping fields: the Philippines' colonial past, contemporary Global Health networks, local politics and government, therapeutic landscapes, people's homes and gardens and the arena of the university. The 'malarias' we played with took on many forms: protectors and oppressors; top policy priorities and things of the past; acute afflictions inside bodies and chronic manifestations of social and community relations; objects of foreign researchers' observations and painful lived experiences for hundreds of Bataraza's citizens. Sometimes, the balls were thrust right upon us, compelling us to take up conscious and deliberative action. Other times, our eyes were off the balls as our bodies unconsciously played on nevertheless. Crucially, even if all the balls were thrown high enough in the sky to disappear, as Danny had put it, the game would continue regardless of whether different objects were placed at its centre, a fresh set of players brought on court or a new collection of prizes made available at the end.

In other words, the people of Bataraza showed me that malaria *was* (un)conscious strategy. As players enacted their daily lives they were positioned, and positioned themselves, in ways that would help them to achieve an array of goals that ranged from winning electoral votes to socialising with friends; dominating foreign countries to attracting customers; establishing a nation to cooling the liver; gaining career satisfaction to preventing the universe being swallowed up whole. As these players were enmeshed in complex ecological, political, social, cultural, material and semiotic conditions, their practices were intimately entangled with various others, including those of non-human actors. This meant that malaria and malaria parasites were consciously and unconsciously embroiled into the mix, which explains why disease and strategic practice were so closely intertwined, or as Singer (2016) put it, why disease is a point of contact between health and 'interest' (ibid., p. 237). Just as with the multiple balls in play, in some cases people's strategic practices were very consciously orientated around malaria, such as when local politicians hailed their success in controlling it, when healers looked for it in bodies or when patients used medicines to try and calm their bodies of its symptoms. At other times, practices were more unconsciously orientated around, or even completely outside, malaria's orbit. They were more focussed on 'civilising' Indigenous Peoples, assuaging the unseen *diwata* in the landscape or on mounting opposition to mining companies. Whether consciously or unconsciously implicated, the disease nevertheless remained entwined along the way—it shaped the trajectory of these strategic relations in specific, albeit ambiguous ways, and was in turn shaped in particular ways itself.

I began this work with a question about how and why it was that malaria both frustrated and facilitated life for the Indigenous Pälawan and what this might tell us about the nature of the disease specifically but also about social relations more broadly. The answers came in the reverse order. In terms of the implications for sociality, I learned that malaria emerged from and was intrinsic to a whole host of strategically orientated social practices that were enacted in as well as around the disease's name, as people worked day-to-day to gain power in different guises in different arenas. In terms of disease, I learnt that its power was not intrinsic or a given, but rather it was moulded alongside these complex webs of relations in which many trajectories and interests were at stake. Power flowed through in more complex formulations than zero-sum scenarios of win versus lose, parasites versus people or sickness versus health. Finally, in terms of the Pälawan, I learnt how it was for these reasons that some were able to harness malaria alongside their strategies to achieve power, such as resisting colonial advances or establishing themselves as legitimate healers. Meanwhile, others were less able to do so when their circumstances or position meant that they lacked the resources or networks necessary to effect change, such as in trying to prevent misfortune in life or adequately punish incest.

These answers yielded yet more questions, namely: what should be done in response? Despite all the heterogeneity, there was one matter upon which everyone I met in Bataraza was agreed—that they wanted to take steps to alleviate the pain, suffering and death surrounding malaria. Given that my contention is that malaria was (un)conscious strategic practice, I suggest that it makes most sense to focus on human practice rather than on malaria alone. Part of my doctoral work involved not just exploring the practices surrounding malaria but also evaluating the impact of an intervention that had the potential to alter them. Specifically, for four months I worked with 44 predominantly Pälawan children aged 9–14 who attended two Elementary schools in Bataraza. I was interested in understanding their lived experience of malaria as well as the role they played in shaping their own and their communities' health. We met weekly in small groups to discuss the photographs that they had taken in response to the question 'What does malaria mean to you?'. The idea was not only to share experiences amongst us but for the children to decide what they wanted, or could, to do to extend this experience to others—their peers, their teachers, their families, their wider community and the health and local government leaders described in this book. My intention was to evaluate the process and impact of this Participatory-Action-Research (PAR) methodology, called photovoice (Wang, 1999; Wang & Burris, 1994, 1997), on children and their immediate families to try to understand if and how it 'worked' to change practice from an anthropological perspective.

In terms of what happened, engaging in photovoice did certainly appear to alter not just children's practices related to malaria but also those of their families (Iskander, 2015a, b, 2019). After weeks of capturing, sharing and discussing images in our groups, children decided to make a range of outputs in order to share their experiences with others. They used their photographs to create exhibitions and banners for their schools; posters and pictorial checklists for their homes; films inspired by their photographs for community screenings; and a series of events for showcasing their experiences and outputs. Through these different formats, children showed each other, myself and their wider community what they did to both prevent and treat malaria; how they kept their bodies healthy and in equilibrium by eating rice and vegetables or were careful not to cool them too quickly with cold baths or coconut water; how they washed their food, boiled their water, took a daily bath and regularly cut their nails to prevent getting dirt inside them; how they cleared their environment of stagnant water, rubbish and dead vegetation to minimise dirty places for mosquitoes to live; how they reduced the chance of getting bitten by keeping carabao close to their houses, repairing and using mosquito nets and slapping insects off their skin; how they took prompt action to deal with sickness in ways ranging from praying to God to going to see Danny in the health clinic; and, finally, how they kept their surroundings and relationships with humans and non-humans beautiful and happy by growing plants and flowers and being respectful, generous and kind. Through participant observation, detailed household surveys and in-depth interviews, I found that as well as the changes to malaria-related practices among children and caregivers, students also learnt new skills, made new friends, felt less shy and more able to communicate with others (Iskander, 2015a, b, 2019). Overall, photovoice seemed to have had an impact on young people's role in shaping their own and others' practices in a more general sense.

In terms of how this happened, I have shown how rather than communicate, gain or pass on knowledge *of* malaria, children generated and circulated bodily knowledge of how they *did* malaria (Iskander, 2019)— of how they (un)consciously practiced it in a broad sense, so to speak. In the process of making photographs, they engaged in, acquired, captured, shared and transformed bodily acts. For example, they mimicked mine and each other's bodies in the process of learning how to use a camera, moving in ways that transformed our manner of being together (ibid.). As they set about taking photographs of their daily lives, they engaged their bodies in the actions described above or imitated them when what they wanted to capture wasn't at their disposal. They created mimetic copies of these practices in the form of images on glossy paper, verbal or written descriptions, moving films and drawings on posters in equally embodied ways and then passed on this practical knowledge by showing (not telling) others. As such, what they reported as having changed the most was not their knowledge or actions to do with malaria but their skills in photography, writing, drawing, public speaking, acting, singing, teaching and so on. As well as propelling bodies into mimetic and creative motion, the process also engaged and elicited emotional bodily responses that they described as 'fun', 'happiness', 'excitement', 'confidence' and 'togetherness'. Teachers, caregivers and community members too reported that children had 'transformed' after the project—they laughed, joked and sang more, were eager to speak up in class, helped around the house and were more confident around new people. Rather than simply being an outcome of the research process or an important way to engage children in the 'serious' business of understanding disease, I contend that 'fun' may have been the mechanism through which photovoice actually made bodies feel—and therefore do—disease differently (ibid.). Finally, because photovoice required the body to interact with a whole host of 'others' from cameras and tripods to parents and policy-makers, practical engagement was interrelational and inter-subjective. The process facilitated and changed relationships (ibid.). It highlighted and reinforced the communal nature of practice and the vast networks that contain it. As such, what this project showed me was that in order to influence (un)conscious practice, what needed to happen was not only that individual participants were to be given the space to consciously think differently about malaria and their practices that directly related to it but, rather, that it was also necessary to give space for collectives of people to unconsciously practice differently and to engage in actions that sometimes only tangentially related to malaria such as singing, acting or helping their parents with chores.

What I have taken from this experience and the experiences that the people of Bataraza shared with me is that 'tackling malaria' is not about malaria, it is about human practice. In contrast to many global and public health campaigns that focus solely on the mechanisms of disease, I suggest we focus on the people who handle it—on the strategies that they pursue, on the power they are trying to obtain and on the tools and networks that they have at their disposal to do so. Malaria has moulded these trajectories in certain and specific ways, it has after all been with us for all of human history, but the power of parasites lies in the practices of people. In terms of how to change the course of human practice and to what end, Welsh (2014) summarises Merleau-Ponty (1996) eloquently when she suggests that we cannot captain bodies like we captain a ship. Even if we wished it to be so, the body can never be made neutral, compelled to stand apart from all the complexity it is enmeshed in in order to choose some kind of more 'appropriate' action. It is always engaged in a non-neutral manner, invested in and connected to the situation it finds itself in, orientated around numerous goals that make any simple kind of agency elusive (ibid.). Freedom is not evidenced by moments of choice, the mental decision to act in one way over another. Rather, freedom is about a 'field', a 'horizon', a 'manner of being in the world'—it is more about the place in which one finds oneself (ibid.). Our understanding of malaria can and should never be placeless and so arguably our interventions should focus more on those places (or fields) in which human practice unfolds—on the conditions that would allow Illaine to keep her pharmacy competitive without having to sell prescription-only drugs when there was none; mean Narcita could be paid for days of work even when she stayed at home due to sickness; enable *Barangay* Captains to retain office without sanctioning the destruction of Pälawan ancestral lands; and help Danny keep his clinic running without having to prioritise malaria at the expense of other issues that threaten the health of Pälawan people. It is unclear how changing the context and these practices would necessarily influence malaria—the relationships are not always so clear-cut as has been demonstrated in this book. However, the point is that attention would be paid to the fact that all these factors (and many more) relate to each other in obscure and murky ways—that the whole is *other than* (not greater than, as is often misquoted) the sum of its parts. It might mean that rather than only try to destroy disease, we would try to relate to it in different ways (Stonington, 2020). As for Danny, sitting on his porch talking about malaria and basketball was the last time I saw him. He died a few weeks later. He left this world before reaching his goal of a malaria-free municipality. In his absence, the game goes on. Without him, malaria remains in all our hands.

References

Bourdieu, P. (1977). *Outline of a theory of practice*. Cambridge University Press.

Iskander, D. (2015a). Parasites, power, and photography. *Trends in Parasitology, 32*(1), 2–3.

Iskander, D. (2015b). Re-imaging malaria in the Philippines: How photovoice can help to re-imagine malaria. *Malaria Journal, 14*(1), 257.

Iskander, D. (2019). How photographs 'empower' bodies to act differently. In A. Parkhusrt & T. Carroll (Eds.), *Medical materialities: Toward a material culture of medical anthropology* (1st ed.). Routledge.

Merleau-Ponty, M. (1996). *Phenomenology of perception* (C. Smith, Trans.). Routledge.

Singer, M. (2016). *The anthropology of infectious disease*. Routledge.

Stonington, S. D. (2020). Karma masters: The ethical wound, hauntological choreography, and complex personhood in Thailand. *American Anthropologist, 122*(4), 759–770.

Wang, C. (1999). Photovoice: A participatory action research strategy applied to women's health. *Journal of Womens Health, 8*(2), 185–192.

Wang, C., & Burris, M. A. (1994). Empowerment through Photo Novella – Portraits of participation. *Health Education Quarterly, 21*(2), 171–186.

Wang, C., & Burris, M. A. (1997). Photovoice: Concept, methodology, and use for participatory needs assessment. *Health Education & Behavior, 24*(3), 369–387.

Welsh, T. (2014). Fat eats: A phenomenology of decadence, food, and health. In T. Conroy (Ed.), *Food and everyday life*. Lexington Books.

Index[1]

---

[1] Note: Page numbers followed by 'n' refer to notes.

© The Author(s), under exclusive license to Springer Nature Singapore Pte Ltd. 2021
D. Iskander, *The Power of Parasites*, https://doi.org/10.1007/978-981-16-6764-0